Vitreoretinal Disease: Clinical Insights and Treatment Strategies

Vitreoretinal Disease: Clinical Insights and Treatment Strategies

Guest Editor

Makoto Inoue

MDPI

Basel • Beijing • Wuhan • Barcelona • Belgrade • Novi Sad • Cluj • Manchester

Guest Editor
Makoto Inoue
Department of Ophthalmology
Kyorin University School of
Medicine
Tokyo
Japan

Editorial Office
MDPI AG
Grosspeteranlage 5
4052 Basel, Switzerland

This is a reprint of the Special Issue, published open access by the journal *Journal of Clinical Medicine* (ISSN 2077-0383), freely accessible at: https://www.mdpi.com/journal/jcm/special_issues/2TCK036MJ4.

For citation purposes, cite each article independently as indicated on the article page online and as indicated below:

Lastname, A.A.; Lastname, B.B. Article Title. *Journal Name* **Year**, *Volume Number*, Page Range.

ISBN 978-3-7258-5853-8 (Hbk)
ISBN 978-3-7258-5854-5 (PDF)
https://doi.org/10.3390/books978-3-7258-5854-5

Contents

About the Editor

Makoto Inoue

Makoto Inoue, MD, PhD, is currently a Professor of Ophthalmology at Kyorin Eye Center, Kyorin University School of Medicine, Tokyo, Japan. He graduated from Keio University Medical School, Tokyo, Japan, in 1989; completed his residency in Ophthalmology at Keio University in 1992; and completed a vitreoretinal fellowship at Kyorin University, Tokyo, Japan, in 1994. Dr. Inoue was a research fellow of Duke Eye Center, Durham, North Carolina, from 1997 to 1999. His research interests are focused on investigating vitreoretinal pathologies and developing new technologies for vitreoretinal surgery, including heads-up surgery with the use of intraoperative OCT.

Journal of
Clinical Medicine

MDPI

Article

Comparison of 27-Gauge to 25-Gauge Vitrectomy in Patients with Tractional Retinal Detachment Associated with Proliferative Diabetic Retinopathy

Hiromi Ohara, Tomohiko Torikai, Jun Takeuchi, Tadashi Yokoi, Takashi Koto and Makoto Inoue *

Kyorin Eye Center, Kyorin University School of Medicine, 6-20-2 Shinkawa, Mitaka, Tokyo 186-8611, Japan; tomohiko-torikai@ks.kyorin-u.ac.jp (T.T.); jun-takeuchi@ks.kyorin-u.ac.jp (J.T.); tadashi-yokoi@ks.kyorin-u.ac.jp (T.Y.); koto@ks.kyorin-u.ac.jp (T.K.)
* Correspondence: inoue-eye@ks.kyorin-u.ac.jp; Tel.: +81-42-247-5511

Abstract: Background/Objectives: To compare the surgical outcomes of 25-gauge (G) vitrectomy to those of 27G vitrectomy for proliferative diabetic retinopathy (PDR) with a tractional retinal detachment (TRD). **Methods:** Eighty-three consecutive eyes of 71 patients with PDR and TRD that underwent initial vitrectomy at the Kyorin Eye Center from June 2021 to August 2023 and were followed for ≥3 months were studied retrospectively. The surgical outcomes of the 10,000 cut/min (cpm) 25G vitrectomy (25G group, 25 eyes) to that of the 20,000 cpm 27G vitrectomy (27G group, 58 eyes) were compared. **Results:** The preoperative PDR status, surgical procedures, and postoperative outcomes were assessed relative to the surgical success. The 25G group had significantly more eyes with severe PDR (p = 0.010), no prior laser photocoagulation (p = 0.027), macular detachment (p = 0.006), and the use of bimanual technique (p = 0.005). However, the operative times and incidence of iatrogenic breaks were not significantly different. The visual acuity improved significantly in both groups at 3 months postoperatively. The primary anatomical success was 88% in the 25G and 97% in the 27G groups (p > 0.05). The risk factors for a postoperative retinal detachment were significantly associated with the grade (p = 0.042) and type of PDR (p = 0.041), the use of perfluorocarbon liquid (p = 0.028), and bimanual techniques (p = 0.017). **Conclusions:** The high anatomical success for both groups for TRD secondary to PDR indicates that both can be used to treat eyes with PDR. The 27G vitrectomy may reduce the need for bimanual techniques.

Keywords: tractional retinal detachment; proliferative diabetic retinopathy; vitrectomy; 27-gauge; 25-gauge, twin duty cycle

1. Introduction

Proliferative diabetic retinopathy (PDR) can progress to vitreous hemorrhages, tractional retinal detachment (TRD), combined tractional and rhegmatogenous retinal detachment (RRD), and neovascular glaucoma [1,2]. Pars plana vitrectomy (PPV) is used to treat these complications, and the Diabetic Retinopathy Vitrectomy Study has reported on the benefits of early PPV [1]. The aims of PPV are to remove the vitreous hemorrhage and the retinal traction, create posterior vitreous detachments, remove fibrovascular membranes (FVMs), and treat areas of retinal ischemia [2]. The degree of surgical difficulty varies considerably and depends on the severity and degree of the PDR [2].

The essential step in PPV is to remove the FVMs, which then reduces the traction on the retina. However, releasing the retinal traction during PPV can also induce bleeding

 https://doi.org/10.3390/jcm14072533

and retinal breaks [3]. The procedures and instruments used during PPV have significantly improved, especially the use of microincision vitrectomy systems (MIVS) [4–6]. The use of intraoperative intraocular pressure (IOP) stabilization systems, wide-angle endo-illumination, and wide-angle viewing systems has also improved the success rate.

Recently, beveled-tip high-speed, dual-blade, twin-duty cycle vitreous cutters have become available. These cutters have improved the vitrectomy procedures, which, in turn, have expanded the pathologies that can be treated by vitrectomy. There has also been an improvement in the outcomes of vitrectomy to treat severe PDR cases [4–14]. Additionally, the use of the 27-gauge (G) system is associated with fewer cases of postoperative low intraocular pressure (IOP) [7,8] and the need for suturing [9–11] compared to the 25-G systems. There are also only minor changes in the corneal topography and astigmatism, which result in rapid postoperative visual recovery [11].

Previous studies comparing the 25G and 27G systems primarily used single-blade cutters. Although the beveled, high-speed, and dual-blade (twin-duty cycle) cutters have been improved, there are only a few reports on using the twin-duty cycle technology for the treatment of PDR [12]. Thus, the purpose of this study was to assess the advantages and risks of using the 27G twin-duty cycle system to treat eyes with PDR. The results were compared to the results of a 25G single-blade cutter system.

2. Materials and Methods

This single-center, observational study was approved by the Institutional Review Committee of the Kyorin University School of Medicine (2403-01). It adhered to the tenets of the Declaration of Helsinki. All of the patients received a detailed explanation of the surgical and ophthalmic procedures, and all signed an informed consent form. All of the patients consented to our review of their medical records and their anonymized use in medical publications.

2.1. Study Population

This was a retrospective study of patients who had undergone 25G vitrectomy with a single-blade cutter at 10,000 cuts per min (cpm; 25G Group, Alcon Laboratories, Inc., Fort Worth, TX, USA) or 27G vitrectomy with a dual blade cutter at 20,000 cpm (27G Group; Alcon Laboratories, Inc., Fort Worth, TX, USA, Figure 1). All surgeries were performed at the Kyorin University Hospital to treat the TRD, followed by PDR between June 2021 and August 2023. All patients were followed for at least 3 months. Patients were excluded if they had a history of PPV, RRD not followed by PDR, and an exudative or traumatic retinal detachment.

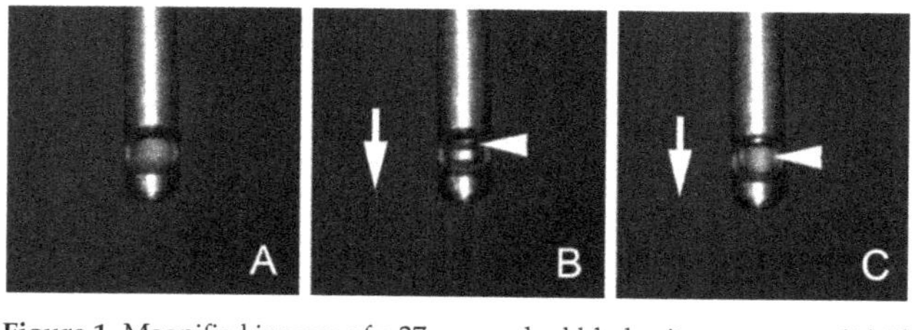

Figure 1. Magnified images of a 27-gauge dual-blade vitreous cutter. (**A**) The opening port of an outer tube is fully opened, and an inner tube of the cutter is located behind the opening port. (**B**) The opening port of the outer tube is closed by the movement of the inner tube forward (arrow). The inner tube has another opening port (arrowhead) that enables fluid or vitreous to be aspirated. (**C**) The opening port of the outer tube is closed by the movement of the inner tube forward (arrow). However, the inner tube has another opening port (arrowhead) that enables fluid or vitreous to be aspirated. This indicates a twin-duty cycle system. On the other hand, a single-blade cutter has no opening port in the inner tube, so when the inner tube is closed, the aspiration is stopped.

2.2. Objectives and Data Collection

The primary outcome was a comparison of the surgical results and the complications of the 25G to the 27G systems. The secondary outcomes were the primary success rates and the identification of factors associated with the success in reattaching the retinal detachment.

The data collected from the medical records were the age at the time of surgery, sex, type of diabetes mellitus, best-corrected visual acuity (BCVA), and IOP (mmHg) at the baseline and at 3 months after the surgery. We also collected information on whether any prior preoperative laser photocoagulation or injections of anti-vascular endothelial growth factor (VEGF) agents had been performed either alone or combined with RRD or neovascular glaucoma, macular detachment, the extent of FVM, and the surgical indications. The extent of the FVM and the surgical indications were determined from the earlier reports [13]. The extent of the FVM was classified as multiple-point adhesions with or without one site plaque-like broad adhesion (Grade 1), broad adhesions in fewer than three sites located from the posterior pole to the equator (Grade 2), broad adhesions in more than three sites located posterior to the equator, or extending beyond the equator within one quadrant (Grade 3), and broad adhesions extending beyond the equator for more than one quadrant (Grade 4) [13].

The surgical indications for PDR included tractional macular thickening, elevation or retinoschisis (Group III), tractional macular detachment (Group IV), and combined traction and RRD (Group V). We injected anti-VEGF agents within 7 days before the PPV in selected eyes [3]. The surgery included the use of 25G or 27G vitrectomy systems, operation time (minutes), use of perfluorocarbon liquid, bimanual technique, incidence of iatrogenic break, and tamponade agent (air, sulfur hexafluoride [SF6], octafluoropropane [C3F8], or silicone oil). We analyzed the optical coherence tomographic (OCT) findings in patients (n = 63) whose preoperative OCT images could be used to evaluate the disruption of the external limiting membrane (ELM) or the ellipsoid zone (EZ), and disorganization of the retinal inner layers (DRIL) of the <1 mm area of the macula. Reoperation due to postoperative retinal detachment was also assessed. For patients who received silicone oil tamponade during the initial surgery, primary surgical success was defined as retinal reattachment after successful removal of silicone oil or under silicone oil without recurrent retinal detachment at 3 months. A final surgical failure was defined as the need for additional surgeries to manage recurrent retinal detachment or the presence of residual silicone oil tamponade at the final follow-up. The decimal BCVA was converted to the logarithm of the minimum angle of resolution (logMAR) for the statistical analyses. Poorer visual acuities were graded as counting fingers, 2.0 logMAR units; hand motion, 2.3 logMAR units; light perception, 3.0 logMAR; and no light perception, 4.0 logMAR.

2.3. Surgical Techniques

All patients underwent PPV using the 10,000 cpm 25G or the 20,000 cpm 27G Constellation vitrectomy systems (Alcon Laboratories, Inc., Fort Worth, TX, USA). The decision on which vitrectomy system to use was the surgeon's preference. The duty cycle is the percentage of time the cutter port is open during a cutting cycle. The maximum cutting rate was set at 10,000 cpm in the 25G group or 20,000 cpm in the 27G group. The aspiration pressure was set at 0–650 mmHg. For posterior visualization, the Resight 700 fundus viewing system (Carl Zeiss Meditec AG, Oberkochen, Germany) was used in all cases. Initially, core vitrectomy was performed, and any vitreous hemorrhage was aspirated. The FVM was removed with the vitreous cutter probe, micro-forceps, micro-scissors, or with bimanual techniques. We removed the epiretinal membrane (ERM) or internal limiting membrane that was made visible by injecting brilliant blue G if patients had ERM or macular traction. Panretinal photocoagulation was performed. Phacoemulsification was performed in patients with lens opacities that affected the intraoperative visibility. Air, 20% SF6, 14% C3F8, or silicone oil was used for tamponade when needed.

2.4. Statistical Analyses

The characteristics of the retina at the baseline and the surgical details were compared between the two groups according to surgical outcomes using χ^2 tests, Fisher's exact tests, or Wilcoxon–Mann–Whitney tests. Dunnett's tests were used to compare the visual acuity preoperatively and at 1 and 3 months postoperatively. The JMP software, version 18 (SAS Inc., Cary, NC, USA), was used for all statistical analyses, and a $p < 0.05$ was considered statistically significant.

3. Results

3.1. Preoperative Demographics and Surgical Procedures

The preoperative demographics and surgical procedures of 83 consecutive eyes of 71 patients are shown in Table 1. Twenty-five eyes in the 25G Group and fifty-eight eyes in the 27G Group underwent vitrectomy. The 25G group had a significantly greater number of eyes with severe PDR type (p = 0.010), no prior laser treatment (p = 0.027), macular detachment (p = 0.006), and use of the bimanual technique (p = 0.005; Table 1). However, there were no significant differences in age, type of diabetes mellitus, preoperative BCVA, preoperative injection of anti-VEGF agents, preoperative ELM and EZ disruptions, and preoperative DRIL. Preoperative anti-VEGF injection was performed on 14 eyes with no significant difference in the PDR grade (p = 0.288) or PDR type (p = 0.332). Thirteen of seventy-seven eyes were phakic, and all thirteen eyes underwent lens-sparing vitrectomy; the other sixty-four eyes underwent phaco-vitrectomy.

Table 1. Characteristics and surgical details of patients with tractional retinal detachment according to primary surgical outcome.

	Total (n = 83)	25G (n = 25)	27G (n = 58)	p Value
Age (years) (median) (range)	50.0 (27–75)	51.0 (27–75)	49.5 (31–69)	0.636 §
Male, n (%)	63 (76%)	19 (76%)	44 (76%)	0.989 †
Type 1 diabetes mellitus, n (%)	4 (5%)	2 (8%)	2 (3%)	0.921 ‡
Preoperative BCVA (logMAR) (median) (range)	1.0 (−0.08–4.0)	1.3 (0.2–4.0)	0.9 (−0.08–2.3)	0.344 §
IOP (mmHg) (median) (range)	15.0 (8–36)	13.0 (9–35)	15.0 (8–36)	0.542 §
PDR grade, n (%)				0.129 ‡
1	10 (12%)	1 (4%)	9 (16%)	
2	35 (42%)	8 (32%)	27 (27%)	
3	34 (41%)	14 (56%)	20 (35%)	
4	4 (5%)	2 (8%)	2 (4%)	
PDR type, n (%)				0.010 *,‡
III	39 (47%)	7 (28%)	32 (55%)	
IV	17 (21%)	10 (40%)	7 (12%)	
V	27 (33%)	19 (33%)	8 (32%)	
Preoperative laser photocoagulation, n (%)	72 (87%)	19 (76%)	53 (91%)	0.027 *,†
Neovascular glaucoma, n (%)	3 (4%)	2 (8%)	1 (2%)	0.183 †
Macular detachment, n (%)	31 (37%)	15 (60%)	16 (28%)	0.006 *,†
Preoperative anti-VEGF injection, n (%)	14 (17%)	4 (16%)	10 (17%)	0.889 †
Preoperative ELM disruption, n (%)	38 (60%)	16 (73%)	22 (54%)	0.135 †
Preoperative EZ disruption, n (%)	47 (75%)	18 (82%)	29 (71%)	0.900 †
Preoperative DRIL, n (%)	49 (78%)	20 (91%)	29 (71%)	0.989 †
Operation time (minutes) (median) (range)	117.0 (38–284)	111.0 (68–188)	117.5 (38–284)	0.976 §
Iatrogenic break, n (%)	53 (64%)	16 (64%)	37 (64%)	0.986 †
Perfluorocarbon liquid, n (%)	28 (34%)	9 (36%)	19 (33%)	0.775 †
Bimanual technique, n (%)	25 (30%)	13 (52%)	12 (21%)	0.005 *,†
Tamponade agent, n (%)	64 (77%)	21 (84%)	43 (74%)	0.315 †

*: $p < 0.05$, †: χ^2 test, ‡: Fisher's exact test, §: Wilcoxon–Mann–Whitney test, BCVA, best-corrected visual acuity; logMAR, logarithm of the minimum angle of resolution; IOP, intraocular pressure; PDR, proliferative diabetic retinopathy; VEGF, vascular endothelial growth factor; ELM, external limiting membrane; EZ, ellipsoid zone; DRIL, disorganization of retinal inner layers.

3.2. Comparisons of Postoperative Outcomes Between 25G and 27G Groups

We used SF6 in 42 eyes, C3F8 in 12 eyes, and silicone oil in 10 eyes as a tamponade. The operation time and incidence of iatrogenic retinal tears were not significantly different between the two groups, despite the fact that the 25G group had more severe cases of PDR (Table 1 and Figure 2). The operation time in both the 25G and 27G groups was significantly associated with the PDR type (p = 0.032, Wilcoxon–Mann–Whitney test), preoperative anti-VEGF injection (p = 0.003), use of perfluorocarbon liquid (p = 0.016), use of tamponade agent (p = 0.001), and complications of iatrogenic breaks (p = 0.001). However, there was no significant difference in the other factors.

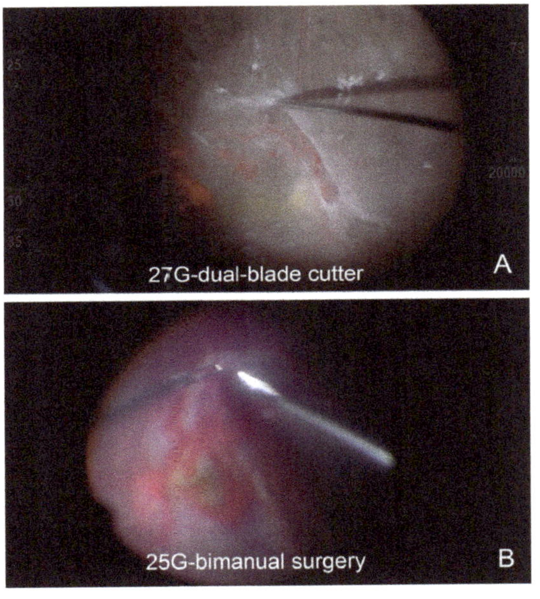

Figure 2. Surgical images during surgery for proliferative diabetic retinopathy with 25-gauge or 27-gauge vitrectomy. (**A**) A fibrovascular membrane is dissected with a 27-gauge dual-blade cutter by inserting the tip of the vitreous cutter beneath the fibrovascular membrane. (**B**) A bimanual technique is used with scissors and forceps of 25-gauge instruments. The fibrovascular membrane is held with the forceps and dissected with scissors in an eye with retinal detachment associated with a tractional membrane complicated by retinal breaks.

The median BCVA at the baseline was 1.0 logMAR units with a range of −0.08 to 4.0 logMAR units. The visual acuity was significantly improved to 0.39 logMAR units (range, −0.08 to 2.3 logMAR units; $p < 0.001$) at 3 months after the surgery. This significant improvement was found in both groups (p = 0.006 in Group 1; $p < 0.001$ in Group 2).

3.3. Primary Success Rates and Risk Factors for Surgical Failure

The primary success rate was 94% for all cases, and it was 88% for the 25G group and 97% for the 27G group (p = 0.153). The grade of the PDR (p = 0.042), the type of PDR (p = 0.041), use of perfluorocarbon liquid (p = 0.028), and bimanual technique (p = 0.017) were significantly associated with primary failure (Table 2). Otherwise, the age, preoperative BCVA, macular detachment, preoperative anti-VEGF injection, preoperative ELM and EZ disruptions, preoperative DRIL, operation time, iatrogenic break, and tamponade agent were not significantly different between the two groups.

Table 2. Characteristics and surgical details of patients with re-detachment.

	Re-Detachment (n = 5)	Primary Attachment (n = 78)	p Value
Age (years) (median) (range)	46.0 (41–74)	50.5 (27–75)	0.792 §
Male, n (%)	4 (80%)	59 (75%)	0.822 †
Type 1 diabetes mellitus, n (%)	1 (25%)	4 (5%)	0.224 ‡
Preoperative BCVA (logMAR) (median) (range)	1.2 (0.5–1.7)	0.9 (−0.08–4.0)	0.826 §
IOP mmHg (median) (range)	10.0 (10–16)	15.0 (8–36)	0.085 §
PDR grade, n (%)			0.042 *,‡
1	0 (0%)	10 (13%)	
2	0 (0%)	35 (45%)	
3	4 (80%)	30 (39%)	
4	1 (20%)	3 (4%)	
PDR type, n (%)			0.041 *,‡
III	0 (0%)	39 (50%)	
IV	2 (40%)	15 (19%)	
V	3 (60%)	24 (31%)	
Preoperative laser photocoagulation, n (%)	3 (60%)	68 (87%)	0.146 †
Neovascular glaucoma, n (%)	0 (0%)	3 (4%)	0.538 †
Macular detachment, n (%)	5 (46%)	26 (31%)	0.577 †
Preoperative anti-VEGF injection, n (%)	2 (40%)	12 (15%)	0.203 †
Preoperative ELM disruption, n (%)	5 (100%)	33 (57%)	0.071 ‡
Preoperative EZ disruption, n (%)	5 (100%)	42 (72%)	0.218 ‡
Preoperative DRIL, n (%)	5 (100%)	44 (76%)	0.271 ‡
Operation time (minutes) (median) (range)	146.0 (96–188)	116.5 (38–284)	0.340 §
25G, n (%)	3 (12%)	22 (88%)	0.153 †
Iatrogenic break, n (%)	1 (20%)	29 (37%)	0.418 †
Perfluorocarbon liquid, n (%)	4 (80%)	24 (31%)	0.028 *,†
Bimanual technique, n (%)	4 (80%)	21 (27%)	0.017 *,†
Tamponade agent, n (%)	5 (100%)	59 (76%)	0.101 †

*: $p < 0.05$, †: χ^2 test, ‡: Fisher's exact test, §: Wilcoxon–Mann–Whitney test, BCVA, best-corrected visual acuity; logMAR, logarithm of the minimum angle of resolution; IOP, intraocular pressure; PDR, proliferative diabetic retinopathy; VEGF, vascular endothelial growth factor, ELM, external limiting membrane; EZ, ellipsoid zone; DRIL, disorganization of retinal inner layers.

3.4. Surgical Failures and Complications

A postoperative retinal detachment was observed in five eyes, and a recurrent retinal detachment caused by the TRD in four eyes (two eyes in the 25G group and two eyes in the 27G group), RRD in one eye (25G group). These five eyes had more severe PDR; four eyes had PDR grade 3, one eye had grade 4, two eyes had type IV PDR, and three eyes had type V. Of the 10 eyes that received silicone oil, 8 eyes had the silicone oil removed, and the retina remained attached. However, a final anatomical success was achieved in 81 eyes (98%), and silicone oil remained in 2 eyes (1 eye in the 25G group and 1 eye in the 27G group).

4. Discussion

The 25G high-speed single-blade cutter and the 27G high-speed dual-blade cutter were used for vitrectomy in eyes with a TRD secondary to PDR. The results showed no significant differences in the operative times or incidence of iatrogenic breaks. Despite the higher proportion of severe PDR cases in the 25G group, the primary retinal reattachment rate, operation time, and incidence of iatrogenic breaks were not significantly different between the two groups. Previous studies have similarly reported no significant differences between 25G and 27G vitrectomies in the primary success rate, operative times, and incidence of iatrogenic breaks [14–16]. The advancements in MIVS, especially with the bevel-tips and 27G vitrectomy probes, allowed more accurate approaches between the FVM and the retina, which had been difficult with the larger cutters [2]. The smaller port size and the more apical location of the port in the 27G cutters enhanced the removal of FVM and reduced the retinal traction during the removal of FVMs. Furthermore, the 27G cutter can function as a multifunctional tool, e.g., as scissors, picks, and back-flush needles, thus reducing the need to change from the cutter to the other instruments [4]. Previous studies indicated that the 27G system had significantly fewer needs for vitreous forceps [10,14] and diathermy coagulation [10], and more efficient FVM removal [10] than the 25G system. The bimanual technique was used significantly less in the 27G group. Despite these advantages, some studies have reported no significant differences in the operative times [10,14,16], iatrogenic breaks [10,14], need for a tamponade [10,16], or reoperation rates [14,16] between the two groups. The nonsignificant differences in the operation times between vitrectomy with 25G single-blade cutters and 27G dual-blade cutters were likely due to the reduced times for instrument changes and increased vitreous aspiration efficiency with the twin-duty cycle system [17,18]. Furthermore, this has been assumed to be because of the design of the inner tube of the dual-blade cutter. The single-blade vitreous cutter has one port on one side, and an inner tube goes back and forth to open and close the port. On the other hand, the dual-blade cutter had an additional inner opening, which led to a constant aspiration [18]. These differences increased the opening time of the port, and the cutting was from both the forward and backward blades of the cutter [18]. The aspiration rates of the twin-duty cycle cutters for balanced salt solution and vitreous have been reported to be significantly higher than those of single-blade cutters at the maximal cutting rate [18]. On the other hand, the fact that the operative time was comparable between the two groups could be attributed to less severe cases in the 27G group that take less time for FVM removal and more time for vitreous cutting. In the 25G group, the opposite reasons applied. The operation time was significantly associated with PDR type, preoperative anti-VEGF injection, use of perfluorocarbon liquid, use of tamponade agent, and complications of iatrogenic breaks. Further randomized and prospective studies are needed.

Our primary reattachment rate was 94% for TRD secondary to severe PDR. This agrees with earlier MIVS reports of 69.2% to 98.9% [13,16,19]. Severe PDR grade and type were significantly associated with a recurrence of retinal detachment. In contrast, previous studies have identified the poor preoperative BCVA factors as younger age, complication of RRD, and silicon oil tamponade as risk factors for redetachment [13,20,21]. Cases involving severe PDR grades or types and extensive proliferative membranes may require more complex surgical procedures, such as perfluorocarbon or silicon oil tamponade [22,23]. In such cases, a postoperative retinal detachment may develop due to iatrogenic breaks, postoperative rhegmatogenous retinal detachment, or persistent or recurrent traction [24].

There are several limitations in our study. First, this was a single-center, retrospective study, and the selection of the PPV system was dependent on each surgeon's preference and the preoperative findings. Thus, there may have been a selection bias and variability in each case. Second, the number of patients was small, and meaningful statistical analyses could not be performed, especially in cases of postoperative retinal detachments. Third, the follow-up period was relatively short. Thus, a prospective study with a larger number of cases is needed to validate the findings of this study.

5. Conclusions

In conclusion, very good primary and final anatomical success was achieved with both the 25G and 27G vitrectomy for TRD secondary to PDR, with significant visual improvements and no difference in operative time or incidence of iatrogenic break. The use of 27G vitrectomy may reduce the use of bimanual techniques, and the 25G vitrectomy is probably a good procedure for severe PDR.

Author Contributions: Conceptualization, H.O., T.K. and M.I.; methodology, H.O. and M.I.; validation, H.O., T.K. and M.I.; formal analysis, H.O., T.T., J.T., T.Y. and T.K.; investigation, H.O. and T.K.; resources, H.O., T.T., J.T., T.Y. and M.I.; writing—original draft preparation, H.O. and T.K.; writing—review and editing, H.O. and M.I.; supervision, M.I.; project administration, H.O., T.T., J.T., T.Y. and T.K. All authors have read and agreed to the published version of the manuscript.

Funding: This research received no external funding.

Institutional Review Board Statement: This study was approved by the Institutional Review Committee of the Kyorin University School of Medicine (2403-01) on 29 July 2024.

Informed Consent Statement: All of the patients received a detailed explanation of the surgical and ophthalmic procedures, and all signed an informed consent form. All of the patients consented to our review of their medical records and their anonymized use in medical publications. The patient's consent for this study was obtained in an opt-out format.

Data Availability Statement: The data presented in this study are available on request from the corresponding author (MI).

Acknowledgments: The authors thank Duco Hamasaki of the Bascom Palmer Eye Institute, University of Miami, Miami, Florida, for discussions and thorough editing of the manuscript. The corresponding author (MI) had full access to all the data in this study and takes responsibility for the integrity of the data and the accuracy of the data analysis.

Conflicts of Interest: H.O., T.T., T.Y.: no disclosures, J.T.: received a research grant from AMO Japan K.K and personal fees (lecture fees) from Novartis Pharma K.K., Santen Pharmaceutical Co., Ltd., Bayer AG, Novartis Pharma K.K., SENJU Pharmaceutical Co., Ltd., Chugai Pharmaceutical Co., Ltd., outside the submitted work. T.K. received research grants from Ellex and Alcon Laboratories, Inc. and personal fees (lecture fees) from Alcon Laboratories, Inc., Novartis Pharma K.K., Bayer AG, Carl Zeiss Meditec AG, Santen Pharmaceutical Co., Ltd., Senju Pharmaceutical Co., Ltd., AMO., outside the submitted work. M.I. received grants from Alcon Laboratories, Inc. and Santen Pharmaceutical Co., Ltd. and personal fees (lecture fees) from Santen Pharmaceutical Co., Ltd., Bayer AG, Novartis Pharma K.K., SENJU Pharmaceutical Co., Ltd., Chugai Pharmaceutical Co., Ltd. Alcon Japan Ltd., Carl Zeiss Meditec, Logic and Design Inc., outside the submitted work.

References

1. The Diabetic Retinopathy Vitrectomy Study Research Group. Early vitrectomy for severe proliferative diabetic retinopathy in eyes with useful vision. Clinical application of results of a randomized trial--Diabetic Retinopathy Vitrectomy Study Report 4. *Ophthalmology* **1988**, *95*, 1321–1334. [CrossRef]
2. Berrocal, M.H.; Acaba, L.A.; Acaba, A. Surgery for Diabetic Eye Complications. *Curr. Diabetes Rep.* **2016**, *16*, 99. [CrossRef]
3. Zhao, L.Q.; Zhu, H.; Zhao, P.Q.; Hu, Y.Q. A systematic review and meta-analysis of clinical outcomes of vitrectomy with or without intravitreal bevacizumab pretreatment for severe diabetic retinopathy. *Br. J. Ophthalmol.* **2011**, *95*, 1216–1222. [CrossRef]
4. Khan, M.A.; Shahlaee, A.; Toussaint, B.; Hsu, J.; Sivalingam, A.; Dugel, P.U.; Lakhanpal, R.R.; Riemann, C.D.; Berrocal, M.H.; Regillo, C.D.; et al. Outcomes of 27 Gauge Microincision Vitrectomy Surgery for Posterior Segment Disease. *Am. J. Ophthalmol.* **2016**, *161*, 36–43.e2. [CrossRef]
5. Yokota, R.; Inoue, M.; Itoh, Y.; Rii, T.; Hirota, K.; Hirakata, A. Comparison of microinsicion vitrectomy and conventional 20-gauge vitrectomy for severe proliferative diabetic retinopathy. *Jpn. J. Ophthalmol.* **2015**, *59*, 288–294. [CrossRef]
6. Sano, M.; Inoue, M.; Itoh, Y.; Hirota, K.; Koto, T.; Hirakata, A. Efficacy of higher cutting rates during microincision vitrectomy for proliferative diabetic retinopathy. *Eur. J. Ophthalmol.* **2016**, *26*, 364–368. [CrossRef]
7. Oshima, Y.; Wakabayashi, T.; Sato, T.; Ohji, M.; Tano, Y. A 27-gauge instrument system for transconjunctival sutureless microincision vitrectomy surgery. *Ophthalmology* **2010**, *117*, 93–102.e2. [CrossRef] [PubMed]
8. Yoneda, K.; Morikawa, K.; Oshima, Y.; Kinoshita, S.; Sotozono, C.; Japan Microincision Vitrectomy Surgery Study Group. Surgical Outcomes of 27-Gauge Vitrectomy for a Consecutive Series of 163 Eyes with Various Vitreous Diseases. *Retina* **2017**, *37*, 2130–2137. [CrossRef]
9. Benzerroug, M.; Marchand, M.; Coisy, S.; Briend, B.; Boussion, B.; Mazit, C. 25-Gauge Versus 27-Gauge Vitrectomy for Management of Vitreoretinal Diseases: A Large Prospective Randomized Trial. *Retina* **2024**, *44*, 991–996. [CrossRef]
10. Liu, J.; Liu, B.; Liu, J.; Wen, D.; Wang, M.; Shao, Y.; Li, X. Comparison of 27-gauge beveled-tip and 25-gauge flat-tip microincision vitrectomy surgery in the treatment of proliferative diabetic retinopathy: A randomized controlled trial. *BMC Ophthalmol.* **2023**, *23*, 504. [CrossRef]
11. Tekin, K.; Sonmez, K.; Inanc, M.; Ozdemir, K.; Goker, Y.S.; Yilmazbas, P. Evaluation of corneal topographic changes and surgically induced astigmatism after transconjunctival 27-gauge microincision vitrectomy surgery. *Int. Ophthalmol.* **2018**, *38*, 635–643. [CrossRef] [PubMed]

12. Nishigushi, R.; Usui-Ouchi, A.; Sakanishi, Y.; Tamaki, K.; Mashimo, K.; Ito, R.; Sakuma, T.; Ebihara, N.; Nakao, S. Outcomes, efficacy and risk factors of 27-Gauge vitrectomy for diabetic tractional retinal detachment in Japanese patients. *Jpn. J. Ophthalmol.* **2025**, *69*, 59–65. [CrossRef]
13. Huang, C.H.; Hsieh, Y.T.; Yang, C.M. Vitrectomy for complications of proliferative diabetic retinopathy in young adults: Clinical features and surgical outcomes. *Graefes Arch. Clin. Exp. Ophthalmol.* **2017**, *255*, 863–871. [CrossRef]
14. Chen, P.L.; Chen, Y.T.; Chen, S.N. Comparison of 27-gauge and 25-gauge vitrectomy in the management of tractional retinal detachment secondary to proliferative diabetic retinopathy. *PLoS ONE* **2021**, *16*, e0249139. [CrossRef]
15. Li, S.; Li, Y.; Wei, L.; Fang, F.; Jiang, Y.; Chen, K.; Yang, X.; Liu, H. 27-gauge microincision vitrectomy surgery compared with 25-gauge microincision vitrectomy surgery on wound closure and need for wound suture and other postoperative parameters in the treatment of vitreoretinal disease: A meta-analysis. *Int. Wound J.* **2023**, *20*, 740–750. [CrossRef] [PubMed]
16. Naruse, Z.; Shimada, H.; Mori, R. Surgical outcomes of 27-gauge and 25-gauge vitrectomy day surgery for proliferative diabetic retinopathy. *Int. Ophthalmol.* **2019**, *39*, 1973–1980. [CrossRef]
17. Inoue, M.; Koto, T.; Hirakata, A. Flow dynamics of beveled-tip and flat-tip vitreous cutters. *Retina* **2021**, *41*, 445–453.
18. Inoue, M.; Koto, T.; Hirakata, A. Comparisons of Flow Dynamics of Dual-Blade to Single-Blade Beveled-Tip Vitreous Cutters. *Ophthalmic Res.* **2022**, *65*, 216–228. [CrossRef]
19. Farouk, M.M.; Naito, T.; Sayed, K.M.; Nagasawa, T.; Katome, T.; Radwan, G.; Abdallah, A.; Elagouz, M. Outcomes of 25-gauge vitrectomy for proliferative diabetic retinopathy. *Graefes Arch. Clin. Exp. Ophthalmol.* **2011**, *249*, 369–376. [CrossRef]
20. Alshaikhsalama, A.M.; Thompson, K.N.; Patrick, H.; Lee, J.; Voor, T.A.; Wang, A.L. Clinical Characteristics and Surgical Outcomes of Patients Undergoing Pars Plana Vitrectomy for Proliferative Diabetic Retinopathy. *Ophthalmol. Retina* **2024**, *8*, 823–831. [CrossRef]
21. Storey, P.P.; Ter-Zakarian, A.; Philander, S.A.; Olmos de Koo, L.; George, M.; Humayun, M.S.; Rodger, D.C.; Ameri, H. Visual and Anatomical Outcomes after Diabetic Traction and Traction-Rhegmatogenous Retinal Detachment Repair. *Retina* **2018**, *38*, 1913–1919. [CrossRef] [PubMed]
22. Hutton, W.L.; Bernstein, I.; Fuller, D. Diabetic traction retinal detachment. Factors influencing final visual acuity. *Ophthalmology* **1980**, *87*, 1071–1077. [CrossRef] [PubMed]
23. Jackson, T.L.; Johnston, R.L.; Donachie, P.H.J.; Williamson, T.H.; Sparrow, J.M.; Steel, D.H. The Royal College of Ophthalmologists' National Ophthalmology Database Study of Vitreoretinal Surgery: Report 6, Diabetic Vitrectomy. *JAMA Ophthalmol.* **2016**, *134*, 79–85. [CrossRef] [PubMed]
24. Dervenis, P.; Dervenis, N.; Smith, J.M.; Steel, D.H.W. Anti-vascular endothelial growth factors in combination with vitrectomy for complications of proliferative diabetic retinopathy. *Cochrane Database Syst. Rev.* **2023**, *2023*, CD008214. [CrossRef]

Journal of
Clinical Medicine

MDPI

Article

Association Between Arch-Shaped Hypo-Autofluorescent Lesions Detected Using Fundus Autofluorescence and Postoperative Hypotony

Yuji Yoshikawa [1,2], Jun Takeuchi [1], Aya Takahashi [1], Masaharu Mizuno [1], Tomoka Ishida [1], Takashi Koto [1] and Makoto Inoue [1,*]

1 Kyorin Eye Center, Kyorin University School of Medicine, 6-20-2 Shinkawa, Mitaka, Tokyo 186-8611, Japan; yuji.yoshi.md@gmail.com (Y.Y.); jun-takeuchi@ks.kyorin-u.ac.jp (J.T.); ayatak1126@gmail.com (A.T.); m-mizuno@ks.kyorin-u.ac.jp (M.M.); tom-oph@ks.kyorin-u.ac.jp (T.I.); koto@ks.kyorin-u.ac.jp (T.K.)

2 Department of Ophthalmology, Saitama Medical University, 38 Morohongo, Saitama 350-0495, Japan

* Correspondence: inoue@eye-center.org; Tel.: +81-422475511

Abstract: Background: Chorioretinal folds are observed after vitrectomy due to ocular collapse caused by low intraocular pressure. The purpose of this study is to investigate the relationship between the postoperative hypotony, chorioretinal folds, and the fundus autofluorescence (FAF) findings. **Methods:** Two-hundred-and-seventy consecutive eyes that had undergone 25- or 27-gauge vitrectomy were examined. The associations between the arch-shaped hypo-autofluorescent lesions in the FAF images and the postoperative hypotony with intraocular pressure (IOP) $\leq$ 4 mmHg were determined on the day after the surgery. **Results:** Arch-shaped hypo-autofluorescent lesions were seen in 4 of the 270 eyes (1.5%), and hypo-autofluorescence was observed in 3 of 14 hypotonic eyes (18.5%). This was significantly more frequent than in the non-hypotony group (0.4%, $p = 0.0004$). Optical coherence tomography showed a loss of the ellipsoid zone and retinal pigment epithelial layer in the region of the arch-shaped lesions. None of the arch-shaped hypo-autofluorescent lesions involved the fovea, and the vision recovered in all cases. The hypo-autofluorescent lesions did not disappear during the 4 to 16 month observation period. **Conclusions:** The postoperative arch-shaped hypo-autofluorescent lesions were associated with postoperative hypotony and RPE damage due to chorioretinal folds. These findings remained even when the IOP was normalized and chorioretinal folds disappeared.

Keywords: chorioretinal fold; fundus autofluorescence; microincision vitrectomy surgery; postoperative hypotony; vitrectomy

1. Introduction

Pars plana vitrectomy is performed for various retinal diseases, and in recent years, microincision and minimally invasive techniques have been used. Microincision vitrectomy surgery (MIVS) with 25-gauge (G) and 27G instruments have been performed with greater safety and reduced complications [1–3]. However, postoperative hypotony is one of the complications after vitrectomy [4–16]. The presence of early postoperative hypotony after 25G pars plana vitrectomy with nonexpansive endotamponade was highly associated with a younger age, prior vitreoretinal surgeries, higher incidence of preoperative ocular hypertension, pseudophakia, silicone oil removal, and use of external diathermy [15]. Bourgault and associates [12] compared the incidence of hypotony after oblique and straight sclerotomies in 25G transconjunctival sutureless vitrectomy. They reported that the incidence of hypotony was not significant different between eyes which had oblique and straight incisions. It has also been reported that the incidence of hypotony was significantly lower in eyes with air or gas tamponade than in fluid-filled eyes [12]. The incidence of ciliochoroidal detachment at sclerotomy sites was detected by anterior segment swept-source optical coherence tomography in 63.3% of 30 eyes with an epiretinal membrane that underwent MIVS during a 1-day observation period [13]. The mean postoperative intraocular pressure (IOP) was significantly lower than the preoperative IOP in eyes with a ciliochoroidal detachment. The mean postoperative IOP was significantly higher in eyes without a ciliochoroidal detachment than in eyes with a ciliochoroidal detachment. The incidence of open sclerotomies was significantly higher in eyes with a ciliochoroidal detachment than in eyes without a ciliochoroidal detachment at 3 h postoperation. Hypotony during the early postoperative period appeared to be associated with a ciliochoroidal detachment at the sclerotomy sites [13].

Earlier studies have shown that in hypotonic eyes with choroidal folds, the retinal pigment epithelium (RPE) is stretched at the crest of the fold and compressed at the trough. These morphological alterations resulted in hyperfluorescence at the crest and hypofluorescence at the trough in the fluorescein angiograms (FA). There is also hyper-autofluorescence at the crest and hypo-autofluorescence at the trough of the fundus autofluorescence (FAF) images [17,18].

We have had cases of postoperative hypotony after vitrectomy that developed arch-shaped hypo-autofluorescent lesions that were coincident with the choroidal folds. However, the relationship between the hypotony and the FAF images has not been determined.

Thus, the purpose of this study was to determine the relationship between the postoperative hypotony and the arch-shaped hypo-autofluorescent lesions that developed after routine pars plana vitrectomy.

2. Materials and Methods

This single-centre observational study was approved by the Institutional Review Committee of the Kyorin University School of Medicine (R04-056). It adhered to the tenets of the Declaration of Helsinki. All of the patients received a detailed explanation of the surgical and ophthalmic procedures, and all signed an informed consent form. All of the patients consented to our review of their medical records and their anonymized use in medical publications.

2.1. Subjects

We reviewed the medical records of 270 consecutive eyes that had undergone routine 25G and 27G pars plana vitrectomy (PPV) between January 2021 and February 2022 and had FAF examinations. The patients were followed for at least 3 months. The procedures used for the vitrectomy were approved by the Kyorin University Hospital Ethics Committee (Reference number; R04-056), and they conformed to the tenets of the Declaration of Helsinki.

2.2. Measurement of Chorieretinal Folds by Optical Coherence Tomography (OCT) and Fundus Autofluorescence (FAF)

The eyes on which a single surgeon (M.I.) had performed the vitrectomy were studied. We collected the age, sex, pre- and postoperative best-corrected visual acuity (BCVA), pre- and postoperative IOP, and axial length from the medical records. OCT images (Spectralis, Heidelberg Engineering, Heidelberg, Germany), infrared scanning laser ophthalmoscopic (SLO) images (Spectralis, Heidelberg Engineering, Heidelberg, Germany), and widefield FAF images (200Tx® or California, Optos Inc., Dunfermline, UK) were also collected. The frequency of arch-shaped hypo-autofluorescent lesions in the FAF images before and after vitrectomy was determined. Then, we determined the association between the arch-shaped hypo-autofluorescent lesions and the pre- and postoperative findings.

2.3. Statistical Analyses

All data are expressed as the means ± standard deviations. A postoperative hypotony was defined as an IOP of ≤4 mmHg on the day after the surgery. Non-parametric tests (Fischer's exact test and Mann–Whitney U test) were used to determine the significance of the differences in the systemic and ocular parameters between the hypotony and non-hypotony groups. All statistical analyses were performed using SPSS (version 28.0; IBM, Armonk, New York, NY, USA).

3. Results

In total, 270 eyes from 270 patients (120 women; 150 men) met the inclusion criteria. The mean age of all participants was 64 ± 14 (±standard deviation) years, and the mean axial length was 25.2 ± 2.1 mm. The pre- and postoperative BCVA was 0.55 ± 0.67 and 0.16 ± 0.47 logarithm of the minimum angle of resolution (logMAR) units, respectively. The pre- and postoperative IOP was 14.6 ± 4.3 and 13.2 ± 6.0 mmHg, respectively. In total, 77 eyes (29%) underwent 25G vitrectomy, and 193 eyes (71%) underwent 27G vitrectomy. Of the 270 eyes, 73 eyes (27%) had an epiretinal membrane, 59 eyes (22%) had a macular hole, 22 eyes (8%) had a dislocation of intraocular lens, 51 eyes (19%) had a rhegmatogenous retinal detachment and/or proliferative vitreoretinopathy, and 28 eyes (10%) had proliferative diabetic retinopathy (Table 1).

Table 1. Demographics of the patients.

Age (years)	64 ± 14
Sex (woman/man)	120/150
Preoperative BCVA (logMAR units)	0.55 ± 0.67
Postoperative BCVA (logMAR units)	0.16 ± 0.47
Preoperative IOP (mmHg)	14.6 ± 4.3
Postoperative IOP (mmHg)	13.2 ± 6.0
Axial length (mm)	25.2 ± 2.1
Arch-shaped hypo-autofluorescent lesions (eyes [%])	4 eyes (1.5%)
Gauge of the vitrectomy (eyes [%])	25G: 77 (29%) 27G:193 (71%)
Pathologies (eyes [%])	
ERM	73 (27%)
MH	59 (22%)
IOL dislocation	22 (8%)
RRD/PVR	51 (19%)
PDR	28 (10%)
Other	37 (14%)

BCVA = best-corrected visual acuity, IOP = intraocular pressure, ERM = epiretinal membrane, MH = macular hole, IOL = intraocular lens, RRD = rhegmtogenous retinal detachment, PVR = proliferative vitreoretinopathy, PDR = proliferative diabetic retinopathy.

The arch-shaped hypo-autofluorescent findings were seen in 4 of the 270 eyes (1.5%) and in 3 of 14 hypotonic eyes (18.5%), which was significantly more frequent than in the non-hypotony eyes (0.4%, p = 0.0004, Tables 2 and 3). In three eyes with markedly low IOP on the day after the surgery, chorioretinal infoldings were observed due to an ocular collapse (Figures 1–4). The FAF images also showed chorioretinal infoldings with the shadowed area corresponding to the trough (valley) of the chorioretinal infoldings. Intravitreal air injection was performed immediately to treat the low IOP. The IOP improved 3 days after the surgery, and the choroidal folds were also improved in all three eyes. The FAF images showed arch-shaped hypo-autofluorescent lesions, which corresponded to the troughs of the chorioretinal folds next to the dark shadowed area.

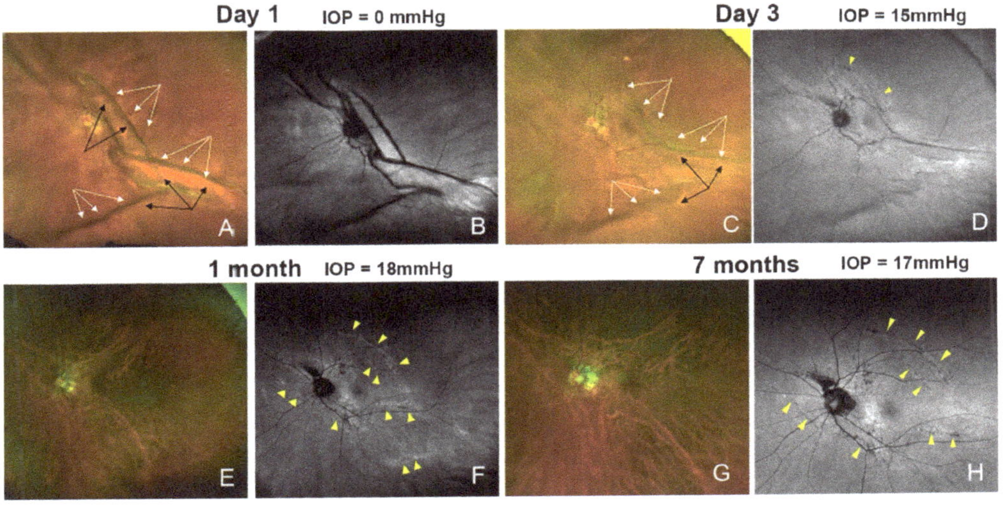

Figure 1. Postoperative fundus photograph and fundus autofluorescent (FAF) images of an eye with an epiretinal membrane in a 64-year-old woman. (**A**) Fundus photograph showing that the eye appears to be deformed by the very low intraocular pressure (IOP) on the day after the surgery, resulting in deformation and severe chorioretinal infoldings with crests (black arrows) and troughs (white arrows). (**B**) FAF image showing the chorioretinal infoldings next to the shadowed area. (**C**) On day 3, the chorioretinal folds are reduced and the IOP is normal. The crests (black arrows) and troughs (white arrows) are flattened. (**D**) FAF image shows arch-shaped hypo-autofluorescent lesions (yellow arrowheads) corresponding to the troughs of the chorioretinal folds with a dark shadowed area next to it. (**E**) At one month, the chorioretinal folds are not present, and vision has recovered to 20/20. (**F**) FAF image shows the arch-shaped hypo-autofluorescent lesions (yellow arrowhead) with hyper-autofluorescent lesions near the hypo-autofluorescent lesions. (**G**,**H**) The hypo-autofluorescent lesions (yellow arrowhead) persisted at 7 months, and were present for 12 months postoperatively.

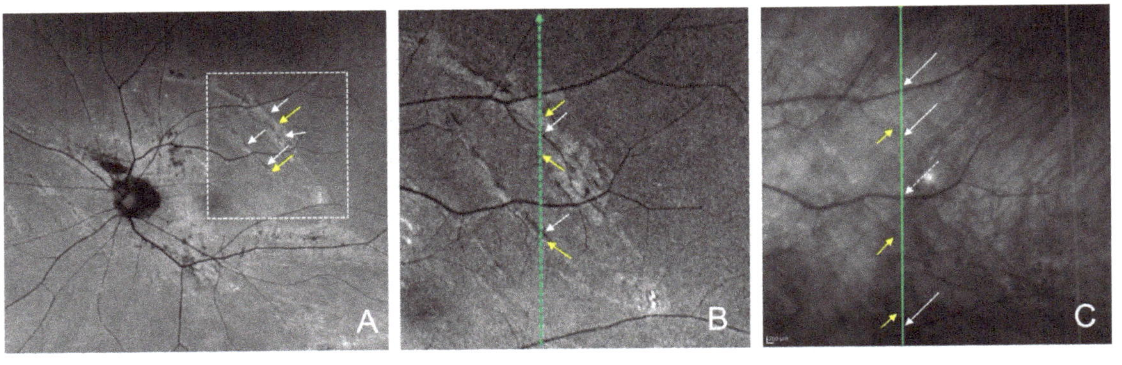

Figure 2. *Cont.*

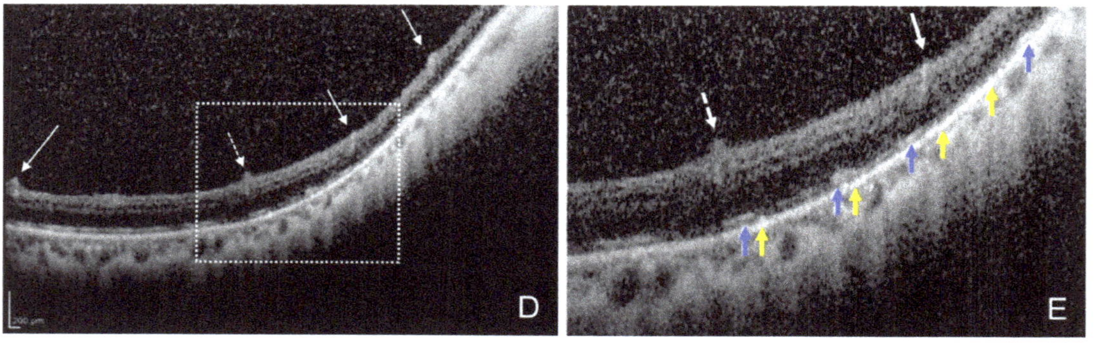

Figure 2. Postoperative fundus autofluorescence (FAF) and optical coherence tomography (OCT) images of the upper chorioretinal fold of the same eye as Figure 1 at one month. (**A**) FAF image and (**B**) magnified FAF image (the dashed square of **A**) show the arch-shaped hypo-autofluorescent lesions (white arrows) with hyper-autofluorescent lesions (yellow arrows). (**C**) Infrared image showing arch-shaped bright lesions (yellow arrows) corresponding to the hypo-autofluorescent lesions in the FAF image. White arrows point to a retinal artery, white dots arrow point to a retinal vein. (**D**) OCT image and (**E**) magnified OCT image (the dashed square of **D**) of a vertical scan (green line of Figure 2B,C) showing the hyperreflective area of the retinal pigment epithelium (yellow arrows), hyperreflective area of the photoreceptor outer segments (blue arrows), and disruption of the ellipsoid zone. White arrows: retinal artery; white dotted arrow: retinal vein.

Table 2. Comparison of cases with or without arch-shaped hypo-autofluorescent lesions.

	Arch-Shaped Hypo-Autofluorescent Lesions (+)	(−)	p-Value
Eyes	4	266	-
Age, years	61 ± 5	64 ± 14	0.573 *
Preoperative BCVA (logMAR units)	0.06 ± 0.05	0.56 ± 0.68	0.050 *
Postoperative Maximum BCVA (log MAR units)	0.19 ± 0.43	0.16 ± 0.47	0.752 *
Pre-IOP (mmHg)	14.3 ± 2.2	14.6 ± 4.3	0.948 *
Axial length (mm)	27.7 ± 3.5	25.1 ± 2.0	0.114 *
Postoperative Hypotony (+)	3 (18.5%)	13 (4.8%)	0.0004 †
Postoperative Hypotony (−)	1 (0.4%)	253 (93.7%)	-

BCVA = best-corrected visual acuity, IOP = intraocular pressure. * Mann–Whitney U test, † Fischer's exact test.

Table 3. Comparison of cases with or without postoperative hypotony.

	Hypotony Group, (n = 16, 5.9%)	Non-Hypotony Group, (n = 254, 94.1%)	p-Value
Age, year	62 ± 11	64 ± 14	0.387 *
Preoperative BCVA (logMAR)	0.33 ± 0.51	0.57 ± 0.68	0.139 *
Postoperative Maximum BCVA (log MAR)	0.11 ± 0.29	0.17 ± 0.48	0.431 *
Pre-IOP (mmHg)	14.6 ± 3.0	14.6 ± 4.3	0.874 *
Axial length (mm)	26.7 ± 2.7	25.2 ± 2.1	0.011 *
Arch-shaped hypo-autofluorescent lesions, eyes (%)	3 (18.5%)	1 (0.4%)	0.0004 †
Gauge of the vitrectomy (eyes [%])	25G: 2 (12.5%), 27G: 14 (87.5%)	25G: 75 (29.5%), 27G: 179 (70.5%)	0.112 †
Pathologies (eyes [%])			
ERM	6 (38%)	67 (26%)	
MH	3 (19%)	56 (22%)	
IOL/lens dislocation	5 (31%)	17 (7%)	
RRD/PVR	0 (0%)	51 (20%)	
PDR	1 (6%)	27 (11%)	
others	1 (6%)	36 (14%)	

BCVA = best-corrected visual acuity, IOP = intraocular pressure, ERM = epiretinal membrane, MH = macular hole, IOL = intraocular lens, RRD = rhegmtogenous retinal detachment, PVR = proliferative vitreoretinopathy, PDR = proliferative diabetic retinopathy. * Mann–Whitney U test, † Fischer's exact test.

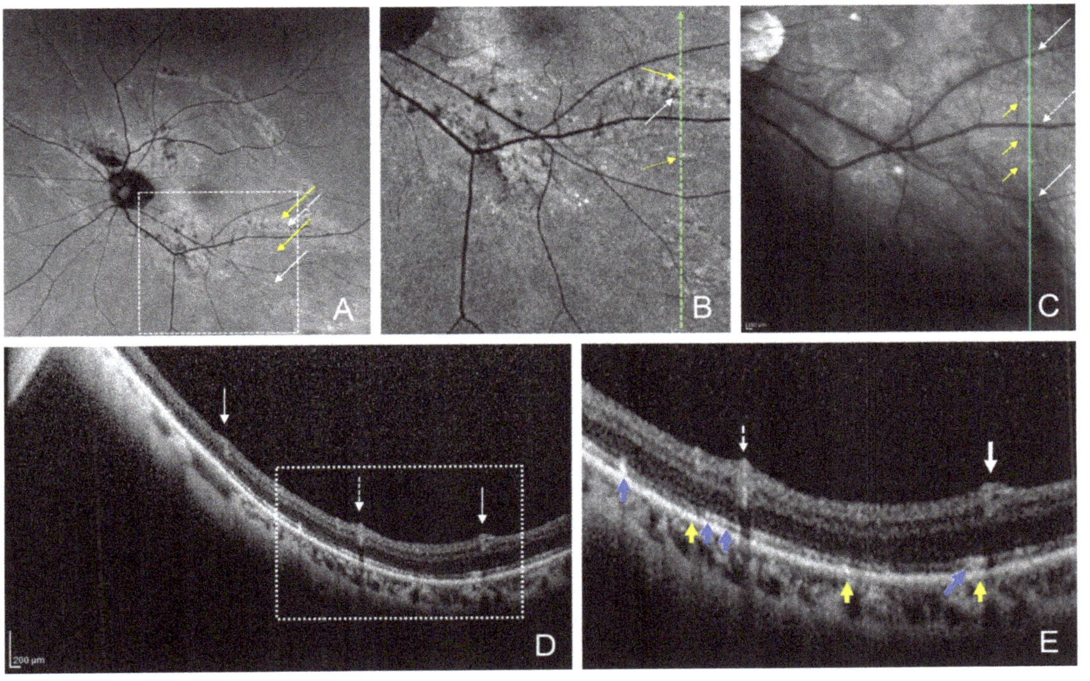

Figure 3. Postoperative fundus autofluorescence (FAF) and optical coherence tomographic (OCT) images of the lower chorioretinal fold of the same eye as Figure 1 at one month. (**A**) FAF image and (**B**) magnified FAF image (the dashed square of **A**) showing the arch-shaped hypo-autofluorescent lesions (white arrows) with hyper-autofluorescent lesions (yellow arrows). (**C**) Infrared image showing bright lesions (yellow arrows) corresponding to the hypo-autofluorescent and hyper-autofluorescent lesions in the FAF image. White arrows point to retinal artery, white dots arrows point to retinal vein. (**D**) OCT image and (**E**) magnified OCT image (the dashed square of **D**) of a vertical scan (green line in Figure 3B,C) showing the hyperreflective area of retinal pigment epithelium and photoreceptor outer segments (yellow arrows), the hyperreflective area of ellipsoid zone band (blue arrows), and disruption of the ellipsoid zone. White arrows: retinal artery; white dotted arrow: retinal vein.

One month after the surgery, fundus examination showed that the chorioretinal folds were not present, but the FAF images showed that the arch-shaped hypo-autofluorescent lesions with hyper-autofluorescent lesions near the hypo-autofluorescent lesions were still present (Figures 1–3) The infrared scanning laser ophthalmoscopic (SLO) images showed that the arch-shaped bright lesions corresponded to the hypo-autofluorescent lesions in the FAF images. The OCT images showed a hyperreflective area of the retinal pigment epithelium and hyperreflective area of photoreceptor outer segments next to the area of the disrupted ellipsoid zone band. The Humphrey 30-2 visual field test did not detect any decreased sensitivity at the site corresponding to the chorioretinal folds in two eyes.

Arched hypo-autofluorescent lesions in the FAF images were observed nasal to the optic disc in all four eyes, and the lesion did not extend to the macula in all four eyes (Figures 1–6). These findings were observed until the last postoperative examination at 16 months. The postoperative BCVA did not differ significantly between the eyes with and without the hypo-autofluorescent lesions (Table 2).

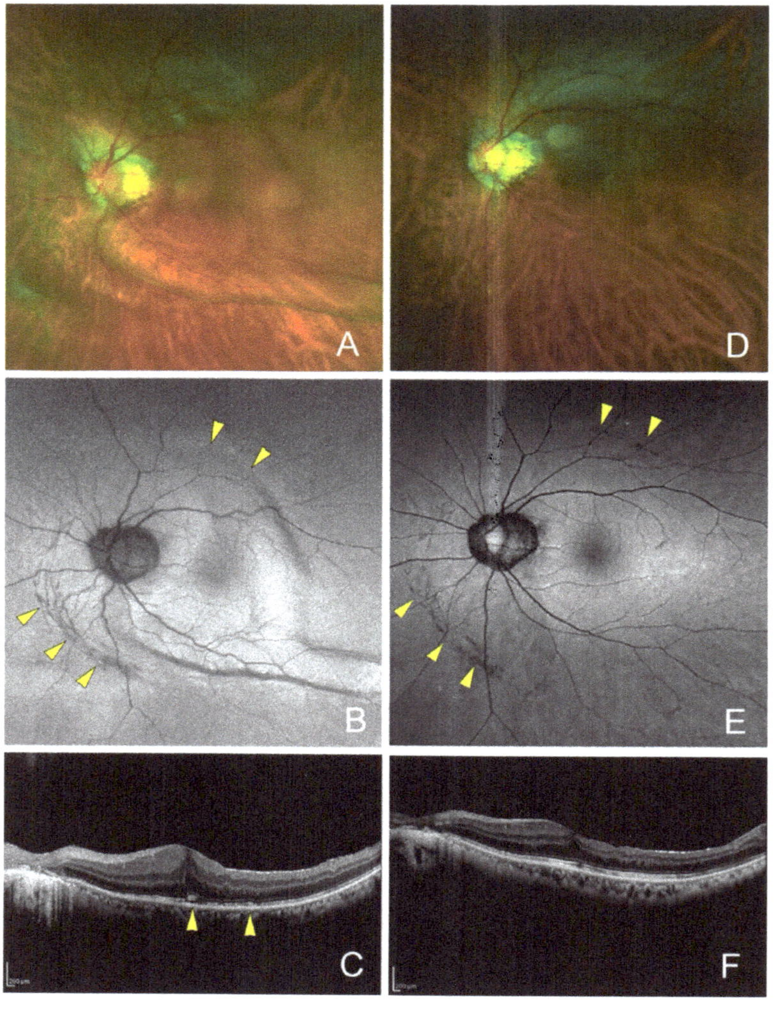

Figure 4. Postoperative fundus photograph and fundus autofluorescent (FAF) images of the left eye of a 63-year-old man with an epiretinal membrane after treatment for a retinal detachment. (**A**) Fundus photograph showing that the eye appears to be deformed by a low intraocular pressure (IOP) of 2 mmHg on day 1 after the surgery. (**B**) Postoperative FAF image on postoperative day 1 showing arched hypo-autofluorescent lesions (yellow arrowheads). (**C**) Optical coherence tomographic (OCT) image of a horizontal section on postoperative 6 days showing the hyperreflective area of the photoreceptor outer segments (yellow arrowheads). (**D**) Postoperative image and FAF image (**E**) at 7 months showing no chorioretinal folds, but persistent arched hypo-autofluorescent lesions (yellow arrowheads). Vision improved to 20/18. (**F**) OCT image showing an absence of the hyperreflective area of the photoreceptor outer segments.

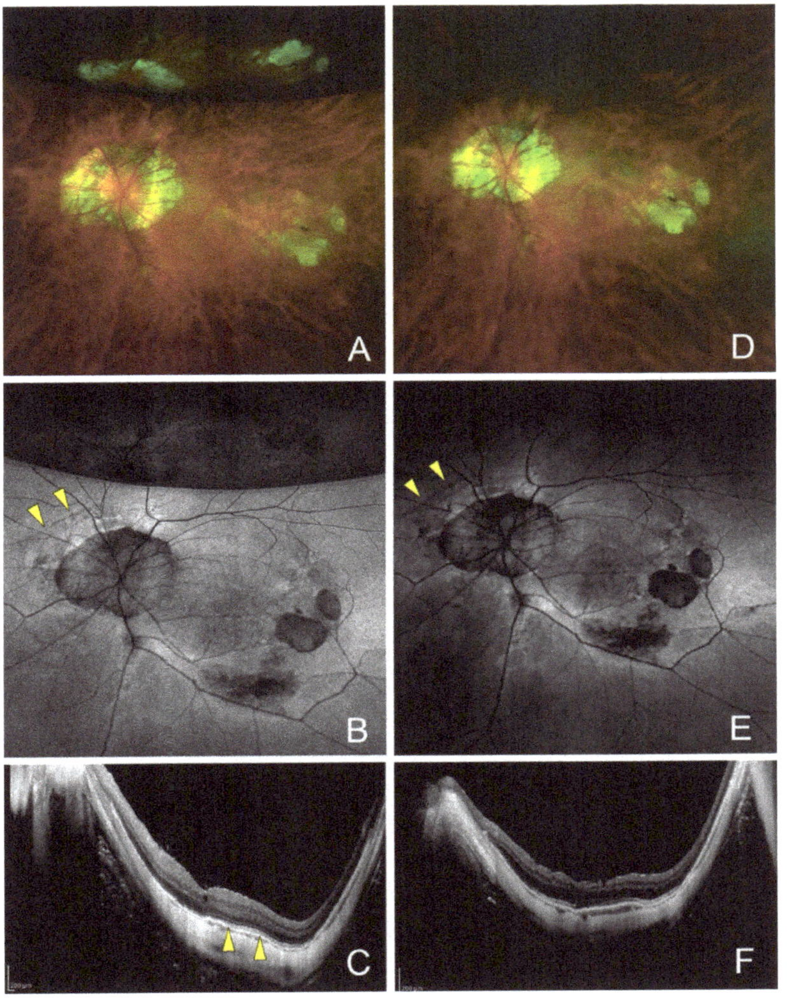

Figure 5. Postoperative fundus photograph and fundus autofluorescent (FAF) images of the left eye of a 64-year-old man with a lamellar macular hole. (**A**) Fundus photograph on postoperative day 7 showing that the eye has recovered from the deformity present on the day after the surgery. Intraocular pressure (IOP) has recovered to 16 mmHg from 3 mmHg on day 1. Intravitreal tamponade air is still present. (**B**) Postoperative FAF image shows arched hypo-autofluorescent lesions (yellow arrowheads) on the nasal side. (**C**) Optical coherence tomographic (OCT) images in a horizontal section on postoperative day 7 showing the hyperreflective elongated area of the photoreceptor outer segment layer (yellow arrowheads). (**D**) Postoperative images and (**E**) FAF image at 4 months after vitrectomy shows the persisted arched hypo-autofluorescent lesions (yellow arrowheads). Vision has improved to 20/20. (**F**) OCT image showing the absence of the hyperreflective area of the photoreceptor outer segment layer.

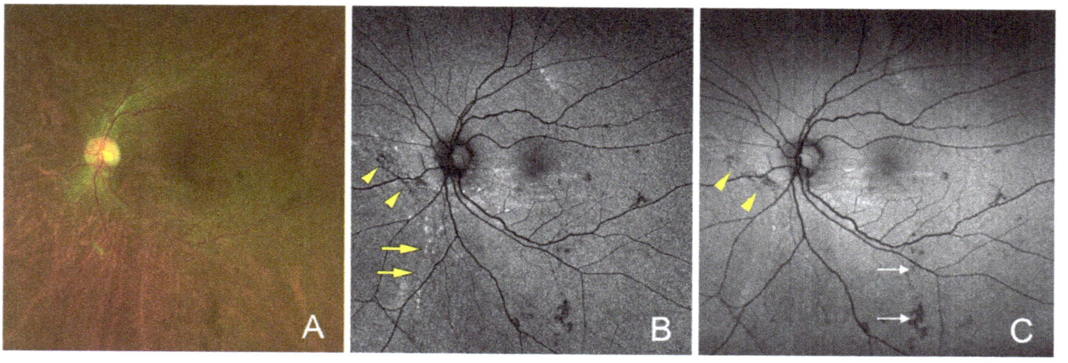

Figure 6. Postoperative images and fundus autofluorescent (FAF) images of the left eye of a 55-year-old man after vitrectomy for a dislocated intraocular lens. (**A**) Fundus photograph on postoperative one month showing no chorioretinal folds. IOP on postoperative day 1 was 12 mmHg. (**B**) FAF image showing arched hypo-autofluorescent lesions (yellow arrowheads) and hyper-autofluorescent lesions (yellow arrows) near and away from the hypo-autofluorescent lesions. (**C**) FAF images at postoperative 7 months showing the persistent hypo-autofluorescent lesions (yellow arrowheads). The hyper-autofluorescent lesions have become fuzzy. Vision was 20/133 due to a previous retinal detachment. Hypo-autofluorescent dots (arrows) were seen before the surgery.

4. Discussion

The arch-shaped hypo-autofluorescent lesions seen in the FAF images after vitrectomy were seen significantly more frequently in the postoperative hypotony group. The sites of these lesions corresponded with the location of the chorioretinal folds, which suggests that they were related to the ocular collapse caused by postoperative hypotony. In addition, these findings persisted for up to 12 months after the surgery, even when the IOP was normalized. The axial length of the eyes in the postoperative hypotony group was significantly longer than that of the non-hypotony group, which indicates that the recovery from early postoperative hypotony was affected by the size of the eyeball. However, the incidence of arch-shaped hypo-autofluorescent lesions was not related to the axial length, but rather to the ocular collapse caused by postoperative hypotony.

In general, hypotony is known to occur after trauma or glaucoma filtering surgery [19,20]. In cases with chorioretinal folds caused by hypotonic maculopathy, the RPE cells are compressed together in the troughs of the folds, resulting in the hyper-autofluorescent lesions in the FAF images. The RPE atrophy occurs at the crests of the folds. These changes result in the hypo-autofluorescent lesions in the FAF images. On the other hand, a posterior staphyloma in highly myopic eyes is known to cause hypo-autofluorescent lesions due to RPE atrophy caused by the expansion of the eyeball [21].

The arched hypo-autofluorescent lesions with hyper-autofluorescent lesions in the FAF images were detected at the troughs of the chorioretinal folds. These folds represent RPE damages due to deformation of the eyeball. In contrast, the hypo-autofluorescent or hyper-autofluorescent lesions in the FAF images were not detected at the crests of the chorioretinal folds. The OCT images revealed hyperreflective areas of the RPE and the photoreceptor outer segments, which represented aggregated RPE cells and the accumulation of photoreceptor outer segments due to RPE damage. The region of the ellipsoid zone in the OCT images also corresponded to the hypo-autofluorescent lesion caused by the RPE damage. The infrared SLO images showed that the arch-shaped bright lesions also corresponded to the RPE damage by their increased reflectivity. These findings in the FAF and SLO images may differ because the chorioretinal folds were displaced and recovered after the recovery from hypotony.

The RPE atrophy was not clearly seen in the OCT images, but the damage of the ellipsoid zone and RPE in the troughs of the chorioretinal fold caused by the extraocular deformation appeared to be more severe than the deformation that usually occurs in hypotonic maculopathy. These changes resulted in the hypo-autofluorescent lesions in the FAF images. There were also cases of arched hyper-autofluorescent lesions located next to hypo-autofluorescent lesions. Hypotonic maculopathy typically occurs after glaucoma surgery. However, the changes in our study were different from the changes seen in hypotonic maculopathy after glaucoma surgery. Possibly, the absence of the vitreous gel made it difficult to maintain the ocular morphology at low IOP, resulting in a more severe ocular collapse and chorioretinal folds that can damage the RPE and photoreceptor cells. Experiments in animal models of myopia have reported that stretching the RPE causes cell expansion and proliferation [22]. The degree of scleral deformation was less at sites away from the chorioretinal troughs, suggesting that the hyper-autofluorescent lesions were caused by RPE aggregation, as seen in hypotonic maculopathy.

These findings did not occur in the macular area and did not affect the postoperative visual acuity. The severe postoperative hypotony on the first postoperative day was treated immediately by the intravitreal injection of air. However, the absence of deformation might be because the location of the optic disc prevented the deformation of the macular area. The chorioretinal folds were described to radiate outward temporally in a branching fashion from the optic disc. However, nasal to the disc, the folds tended to be arranged concentrically by the traction exerted nasally by the optic nerve fibres as they moved [23,24]. One of the four eyes with the postoperative arch-shaped hypo-autofluorescent lesions did not have low IOP the day after the surgery, and no retinal choroidal folds were seen on fundus examination on the next day. The reason for this is not clear, but it is possible that the eye had low IOP immediately after surgery and the IOP had recovered on the next day.

Our study has several limitations. First, the very small number of eyes studied and the retrospective nature limited the strength of the conclusions that can be made. Second, the number of the patients with choroidal fold was too few to perform statistical analyses of findings of the FAF and OCT images. Third, the follow-up period may be too short to make a conclusion to evaluate the eventual outcome of hyper-autofluorescent and hypo-autofluorescent lesions.

5. Conclusions

In conclusion, postoperative arch-shaped hypo-autofluorescent lesions were associated with the postoperative hypotony and RPE damage due to the chorioretinal folds. These changes remained even after the IOP recovered and the chorioretinal folds disappeared.

Author Contributions: Conceptualization, Y.Y., M.I. and T.K.; methodology, Y.Y. and M.I.; validation, Y.Y., M.I. and T.K.; formal analysis, Y.Y., J.T., A.T., T.I. and M.I.; investigation. Y.Y. and M.I.; resources, Y.Y. and M.I.; data curation, Y.Y., J.T., A.T., M.M., T.I. and M.I.; writing—original draft preparation, M.I. and T.K.; writing—review and editing, Y.Y. and M.I.; supervision, T.K.; project administration, Y.Y., J.T., A.T., T.I. and M.I. All authors have read and agreed to the published version of the manuscript.

Funding: This research received no external funding.

Institutional Review Board Statement: This study was approved by the Institutional Review Committee of the Kyorin University School of Medicine (R04-056) on 19 July, 2022.

Informed Consent Statement: All of the patients received a detailed explanation of the surgical and ophthalmic procedures and all signed an informed consent form. All of the patients consented to our review of their medical records and their anonymized use in medical publications. The patient consent of this study was obtained in an opt-out format.

Data Availability Statement: The data presented in this study are available on request from the corresponding author (M.I.).

Acknowledgments: The authors thank Duco Hamasaki of the Bascom Palmer Eye Institute, University of Miami, Miami, Florida, for discussions and thorough editing of the manuscript. The corresponding author (M.I.) had full access to all the data in the study and takes responsibility for the integrity of the data and the accuracy of the data analysis.

Conflicts of Interest: Y.Y.: Personal fees (lecture fees) from Novartis Pharma K.K., Bayer AG, Carl Zeiss Meditec AG, Novartis Pharma K.K., KOWA, AMO., and Chugai Pharmaceutical Co., Ltd., outside the submitted work. J.T.: Research grant from AMO Japan K.K and lecture fees from Novartis Pharma K.K., Santen Pharmaceutical Co., Ltd., Bayer AG, SENJU Pharmaceutical Co., Ltd., Chugai Pharmaceutical Co., Ltd., outside the submitted work. A.T.: No disclosure. MM: Research grants from Alcon Laboratories, Inc., and personal fees (lecture fees) from Alcon Laboratories, Inc., Santen Pharmaceutical Co., Ltd., outside the submitted work. TI: Personal fees (lecture fees) from Nikon Co., Ltd., Santen Pharmaceutical Co., Ltd. TK: Research grants from Alcon Laboratories, Inc., and Ellex, and personal fees (lecture fees) from Alcon Laboratories, Inc., Novartis Pharma K.K., Bayer AG, Carl Zeiss Meditec AG, Novartis Pharma K.K., Santen Pharmaceutical Co., Ltd., and Senju Pharmaceutical Co., Ltd. AMO., outside the submitted work. MI: Research grants from Alcon Laboratories, Inc., and Santen Pharmaceutical Co., Ltd. and personal fees (lecture fees) from Alcon Laboratories, Inc., Novartis Pharma K.K., Bayer AG, Carl Zeiss Meditec AG, Novartis Pharma K.K., Santen Pharmaceutical Co., Ltd., and Senju Pharmaceutical Co., Ltd. AMO, Logitec and Design, outside the submitted work.

References

1. Yoon, Y.H.; Kim, D.S.; Kim, J.G.; Hwang, J.U. Sutureless vitreoretinal surgery using a new 25-gauge transconjunctival system. *Ophthalmic Surg. Lasers Imaging* **2006**, *37*, 12–19. [CrossRef] [PubMed]
2. Oshima, Y.; Wakabayashi, T.; Sato, T.; Ohji, M.; Tano, Y. A 27-gauge instrument system for transconjunctival sutureless microincision vitrectomy surgery. *Ophthalmology* **2010**, *117*, 93–102.e102. [CrossRef]
3. Thompson, J.T. Advantages and limitations of small gauge vitrectomy. *Surv. Ophthalmol.* **2011**, *56*, 162–172. [CrossRef]
4. Williams, B.K.; Chang, J.S.; Flynn, H.W. Optical coherence tomography imaging of chorioretinal folds associated with hypotony maculopathy following pars plana vitrectomy. *Int. Med. Case Rep. J.* **2015**, *8*, 199–203. [CrossRef]
5. Inoue, M.; Shinoda, K.; Shinoda, H.; Kawamura, R.; Suzuki, K.; Ishida, S. Two-step oblique incision during 25-gauge vitrectomy reduces incidence of postoperative hypotony. *Clin. Exp. Ophthalmol.* **2007**, *35*, 693–696. [CrossRef] [PubMed]
6. Byeon, S.H.; Lew, Y.J.; Kim, M.; Kwon, O.W. Wound leakage and hypotony after 25-gauge sutureless vitrectomy: Factors affecting postoperative intraocular pressure. *Ophthalmic Surg. Lasers Imaging* **2008**, *39*, 94–99. [CrossRef] [PubMed]
7. Hsu, J.; Chen, E.; Gupta, O.; Fineman, M.S.; Garg, S.J.; Regillo, C.D. Hypotony after 25-gauge vitrectomy using oblique versus direct cannula insertions in fluid-filled eyes. *Retina* **2008**, *28*, 937–940. [CrossRef] [PubMed]
8. Acar, N.; Kapran, Z.; Unver, Y.B.; Altan, T.; Ozdogan, S. Early postoperative hypotony after 25-gauge sutureless vitrectomy with straight incisions. *Retina* **2008**, *28*, 545–552. [CrossRef] [PubMed]
9. Woo, S.J.; Park, K.H.; Hwang, J.M.; Kim, J.H.; Yu, Y.S.; Chung, H. Risk factors associated with sclerotomy leakage and postoperative hypotony after 23-gauge transconjunctival sutureless vitrectomy. *Retina* **2009**, *29*, 456–463. [CrossRef] [PubMed]
10. Bamonte, G.; Mura, M.; Stevie Tan, H. Hypotony after 25-gauge vitrectomy. *Am. J. Ophthalmol.* **2011**, *151*, 156–160. [CrossRef] [PubMed]
11. Fabian, I.D.; Moisseiev, J. Sutureless vitrectomy: Evolution and current practices. *Br. J. Ophthalmol.* **2011**, *95*, 318–324. [CrossRef] [PubMed]
12. Bourgault, S.; Tourville, E. Incidence of postoperative hypotony in 25-gauge vitrectomy: Oblique versus straight sclerotomies. *Can. J. Ophthalmol.* **2012**, *47*, 21–23. [CrossRef] [PubMed]
13. Yamane, S.; Inoue, M.; Arakawa, A.; Kadonosono, K. Early postoperative hypotony and ciliochoroidal detachment after microincision vitrectomy surgery. *Am. J. Ophthalmol.* **2012**, *153*, 1099–1103.e1. [CrossRef] [PubMed]
14. Gupta, N.; Punjabi, O.S.; Steinle, N.C.; Singh, R.P. Rate of hypotony following 25-gauge pars plana vitrectomy. *Ophthalmic Surg. Lasers Imaging Retina* **2013**, *44*, 155–159. [CrossRef] [PubMed]
15. Mimouni, M.; Abualhasan, H.; Derman, L.; Feldman, A.; Mazzawi, F.; Barak, Y. Incidence and Risk Factors for Hypotony after 25-Gauge Pars Plana Vitrectomy with Nonexpansile Endotamponade. *Retina* **2020**, *40*, 41–46. [CrossRef] [PubMed]
16. Ung, C.; Yonekawa, Y.; Chung, M.M.; Berrocal, A.M.; Kusaka, S.; Oshima, Y.; Chan, R.V.P.; Inoue, M.; Read, S.P.; Kuriyan, A.E.; et al. 27-Gauge Pars Plana/Plicata Vitrectomy for Pediatric Vitreoretinal Surgery. *Retina* **2023**, *43*, 238–242. [CrossRef] [PubMed]
17. Gass, J.D.M. Hypotony maculopathy. In *Contemporary Ophthalmology*; Goldfreed Bellows, J., Ed.; Honoring Sir Stewart Duke-Elder; Williams & Wilkins: Baltimore, MD, USA, 1972; pp. 343–366.
18. Agawal, A. *Gass's Atlas of Macular Disease*, 5th ed.; Saunders: Amsterdam, The Netherlands, 2011; Volume 2, pp. 266–267.
19. Wang, Q.; Thau, A.; Levin, A.V.; Lee, D. Ocular hypotony: A comprehensive review. *Surv. Ophthalmol.* **2019**, *64*, 619–638. [CrossRef]
20. Jampel, H.D.; Pasquale, L.R.; Dibernardo, C. Hypotony maculopathy following trabeculectomy with mitomycin C. *Arch. Ophthalmol.* **1992**, *110*, 1049–1050. [CrossRef] [PubMed]

21. Shinohara, K.; Moriyama, M.; Shimada, N.; Tanaka, Y.; Ohno-Matsui, K. Myopic stretch lines: Linear lesions in fundus of eyes with pathologic myopia that differ from lacquer cracks. *Retina* **2014**, *34*, 461–469. [CrossRef]
22. Lin, T.; Grimes, P.A.; Stone, R.A. Expansion of the retinal pigment epithelium in experimental myopia. *Vision Res.* **1993**, *33*, 1881–1885. [CrossRef]
23. Bullock, J.D.; Egbert, P.R. The origin of choroidal folds a clinical, histopathological, and experimental study. *Doc. Ophthalmol.* **1974**, *37*, 261–293. [CrossRef] [PubMed]
24. Bullock, J.D.; Egbert, P.R. Experimental choroidal folds. *Am. J. Ophthalmol.* **1974**, *78*, 618–623. [CrossRef] [PubMed]

Journal of
Clinical Medicine

MDPI

Article

Basal Linear Deposit: Normal Physiological Ageing or a Defining Lesion of Age-Related Macular Degeneration?

Akshaya Lakshmi Thananjeyan [1,2], Jennifer Arnold [3], Mitchell Lee [4,5], Cheryl Au [5,6], Victoria Pye [4,5], Michele C. Madigan [7,8] and Svetlana Cherepanoff [4,5,6,*]

1 St. Vincent's Hospital, Victoria Street, Darlinghurst, NSW 2010, Australia
2 School of Medicine, University of Sydney, Camperdown, NSW 2006, Australia
3 Marsden Eye Specialists, Parramatta, NSW 2150, Australia
4 School of Clinical Medicine, University of NSW, Sydney, NSW 2052, Australia
5 Anatomical Pathology, St Vincent's Hospital, Darlinghurst, NSW 2010, Australia
6 School of Medicine, University of Notre Dame, Sydney, NSW 2008, Australia
7 Optometry and Vision Science, University of New South Wales (UNSW), Sydney, NSW 2052, Australia
8 Save Sight Institute, University of Sydney, Sydney, NSW 2000, Australia
* Correspondence: svetlana.cherepanoff@svha.org.au; Tel.: +61-2-8382-9168

Abstract: Objective: To determine if basal linear deposit (BLinD) is a specific lesion of age-related macular degeneration (AMD). **Methods:** The cohort was selected from a clinically and histopathologically validated archive (Sarks Archive) and consisted of 10 *normal* eyes (age 55–80 years) without any macular basal laminar deposit (BLamD) (Sarks Group I) and 16 *normal aged* eyes (age 57–88 years) with patchy BLamD (Sarks Group II). Only eyes with in vivo fundus assessment and corresponding high-resolution transmission electron microscopy (TEM) micrographs of the macula were included. Semithin sections and fellow-eye paraffin sections were additionally examined. BLinD was defined as a diffuse layer of electron-lucent vesicles external to the retinal pigment epithelium (RPE) basement membrane by TEM and was graded as follows: (i) Grade 0, absence of a continuous layer; (ii) Grade 1, a continuous layer up to three times the thickness of the RPE basement membrane (0.9 µm); (iii) Grade 2, a continuous layer greater than 0.9 µm. Bruch's membrane (BrM) hyalinisation and RPE abnormalities were determined by light microscopic examination of corresponding semithin and paraffin sections. **Results:** BLinD was identified in both *normal* (30%) and *normal aged* (62.5%) eyes. BLinD was thicker in *normal aged* eyes ($p = 0.045$; 95% CI 0.04–3.4). BLinD thickness positively correlated with both the degree of BrM hyalinisation ($p = 0.049$; 95% CI 0.05–2.69) and increasing microscopic RPE abnormalities ($p = 0.022$; 95% CI 0.188–2.422). RPE abnormalities were more likely to be observed in eyes with increased BrM hyalinisation ($p = 0.044$; 95% CI 0.61–4.319). **Conclusions:** BLinD is most likely an age-related deposit rather than a specific lesion of AMD. Its accumulation is associated with increasing BrM hyalinisation and microscopic RPE abnormalities, suggesting a relationship with dysregulated RPE metabolism and/or transport.

Keywords: age-related macular degeneration; basal linear deposit; basal laminar deposit; ageing

1. Introduction

Age-related macular degeneration (AMD) is a clinically diagnosed disease. Upon fundus ophthalmoscopy, early and intermediate AMD is defined by the presence of soft drusen, with or without pigment changes, whereas late AMD is defined by the presence of geographic atrophy and/or macular neovascularisation (advanced AMD) [1]. Sarks [2] was the first to document the continuum of specific histological changes that accompany each stage of AMD in a large cohort of clinically validated eyes. A continuous and diffuse layer of sub-retinal pigment epithelium (RPE) basal laminar deposit (BLamD) was shown to be the defining histological lesion of AMD. A second diffuse deposit, basal linear deposit (BLinD), was later revealed by transmission electron microscopy (TEM) to be present in all eyes with AMD [3]. BLinD appears as electron-lucent vesicles that accumulate in the inner collagenous zone (ICZ) of Bruch's membrane (BrM), external to the RPE basement membrane. Because BLinD is seen in continuity with soft drusen [4] and is composed of similar electron-lucent vesicles, it is considered a soft drusen precursor [5].

There is extensive evidence that the lipid content within BrM increases with age [6]. There is also substantial evidence that the electron-lucent vesicles that comprise BLinD and soft drusen are lipid-rich [7,8]. Subsequent histological and ultrastructural investigations showed that a BLinD-like deposit could also be found in younger eyes without AMD [4]. These observations raise an important question: is BLinD a specific AMD lesion or is it associated with normal ageing?

One of the difficulties in reconciling published findings to date is the lack of a universal definition of BLinD. The study cohorts on which observations have been based were mixed, with mostly small sample sizes and without in vivo clinical validation. This limits the clinical and histological correlation of identified markers. To address this question, we studied a clinically and histologically validated archive of 10 normal and 16 normal aged human eyes. Using a standardised definition of BLinD, we measured its thickness in electron micrographs and correlated our findings to age as well as light microscopic evaluation of BrM hyalinisation and RPE abnormalities.

2. Materials and Methods

2.1. Ethics

The study protocol was approved by the St Vincent's Hospital Human Research Ethics Committee (REF: 2021/ETH01147) and was monitored by the St Vincent's Hospital Sydney Research Office. Archival records were accessed for research from January to December 2023. Authors did not have access to sufficient information to identify participants during or after data collection.

2.2. Cohort

The Sarks archive consists of over 600 eyes obtained from 1967 to 1995 from over 350 prospectively consenting patients, each with detailed clinical annotations and histological assessment. During the clinical assessment, the best corrected distance visual acuity, fundus assessment, medical history and other intra-ocular findings [2] were documented. In vivo fundus photography was captured when possible. *Post-mortem*, macular histology was assessed by light microscopy. TEM assessment was also performed in most cases on fellow eyes. In vivo fundus findings and clinical progression were correlated with detailed histological and ultrastructural analyses.

2.3. Sarks Histological AMD Grading

Sarks [2] was the first to define ageing and AMD as a continuum of histological changes in a large cohort of clinically validated human eyes. Group I (normal) eyes have no macular BLamD and have a normal fundus. Group II (normal aged) eyes contain patchy, macular BLamD. Group III (early AMD) eyes have a continuous (at least 250 μm), thin (less than half the height of an RPE cell) layer of macular BLamD. The presence of continuous BLamD marks the histological threshold of AMD. Group IV (intermediate AMD) eyes are characterised by continuous, thick (greater than half the height of an RPE cell) macular BLamD, corresponding to the presence of early and intermediate AMD upon fundus examination. Group V eyes are defined by the presence of geographic atrophy and Group VI by disciform scar formation.

2.4. Cohort Inclusion and Exclusion Criteria

Eyes from the Sarks Archive were selected if they met the following inclusion criteria: (i) Group I (normal; no macular BLamD) and Group II (normal aged; patchy macular BLamD); (ii) at least two TEM images of the macula available for assessment; (iii) corresponding macular resin semithin sections for light microscopic evaluation and (iv) well-documented in vivo fundus findings. Cases with paraffin sections of the fellow eye were prioritised for inclusion. Eyes with any macular pathology were excluded. Normal clinical fundus examination findings were confirmed by a review of the clinical notes and, where available, in vivo fundus photographs. Light microscopic review of semithin resin sections and picro-Mallory-stained paraffin sections was undertaken to confirm (i) the absence of AMD, defined by the absence of continuous macular BLamD and (ii) the absence of any other microscopic macular pathology.

2.5. Light and Electron Microscopy

Eyes prepared for TEM were fixed in 2.5% glutaraldehyde in 0.1 M cacodylate buffer, and the macula and optic disc were punched out using an 8 mm corneal trephine [9,10]. After the retina and choroid were dissected away, the tissue was subdivided into blocks and washed in fresh cacodylate buffer, then postfixed in 2% osmium tetroxide in 0.1 M cacodylate buffer. This was followed by 2% uranyl acetate staining. Next, tissue blocks were dehydrated through graded alcohols and acetone, before being embedded in Spurrs low-viscosity resin and cured at 60 °C for 8 h. Semithin 0.5 μm sections were cut and stained with toluidine blue. Ultrastructural areas of interest were identified on semithin resin sections and examined by TEM (Philips 300 Electron Microscope; Eindhoven, The Netherlands) at an accelerating voltage of 80 Kv. TEM micrographs were examined after digital scanning.

Paraffin section methods, described previously [2], were as follows: after fixation in neutral buffered formalin and paraffin embedding, the pupil-to-optic nerve block was sectioned at 8 μm thickness through the macula. Every 10th paraffin section was stained with picro-Mallory trichrome. Coverslipped glass slides of resin and paraffin sections were digitally scanned for microscopic review and data collection.

2.6. Bruch Membrane Hyalinisation

BrM hyalinisation was graded using a scale previously defined by Sarks [2] and later validated by van der Schaft et al. [11]. Briefly, Grade 1 hyalinisation does not extend beyond BrM; Grade 2 hyalinisation reaches the intercapillary pillars; Grade 3 hyalinisation extends through the intercapillary pillars entirely and Grade 4 hyalinisation encircles the choriocapillaries.

2.7. Basal Linear Deposit: Definition

The term "basal linear deposit" was originally used to describe what is now understood to be BLamD, a diffuse, aberrant basement membrane-like deposit *internal* to the RPE basement membrane that is readily identifiable upon *light microscopic* examination of *paraffin sections* after histological staining [2,12]. The distinct properties of BLamD and BLinD only became apparent with the routine availability of TEM. BLinD was first defined in published literature as a layer of electron-lucent vesicles external to the RPE basement membrane using TEM [13]. It was further defined as the precursor lesion for soft drusen in 1994 [14] and subsequently confirmed to be present in all eyes, with histological evidence of early AMD defined as a continuous layer of macular BLamD [3]. There are no published criteria for defining BLinD in terms of thickness or extent in tissue cross-sections. In the absence of published consensus criteria, we defined BLinD as a diffuse layer of electron-lucent vesicles external to the RPE basement membrane that is at least the thickness of the RPE basement membrane (approximately 0.3 μm) [15]. Here, we use the term "electron-lucent vesicles" purely as an ultrastructural morphological descriptor without any functional or biochemical inferences. This deposit was classified as BLinD only when it was seen spanning the entirety of a TEM photograph at low magnification (13.5 × 1000) (approximately 9 μm). The maximum thickness of BLinD in each eye was recorded and graded into the following categories: (i) less than 0.3 μm (Grade 0); (ii) up to 3 × 0.3 μm (Grade 1); and (iii) greater than 3 × 0.3 μm (Grade 2). Three other histological landmarks were used to confirm BLinD thickness: (i) the diameter of a red blood cell within the choriocapillaris, approximately 8 μm [16]; (ii) the diameter of a macular RPE nucleus, approximately 3–12 μm [17]; and (iii) the height of a macular RPE cell, approximately 14 μm [18].

2.8. Imaging and Scanning

Coverslipped glass slides of stained paraffin and resin semithin sections were scanned using an Olympus Slideview VS200 (Olympus Life Science; Tokyo, Japan), a high throughput brightfield and fluorescent slide scanner. The 60×/1.42 oil objective and brightfield imaging mode were used for scanning all slides. Once scanned, slides were assessed using the OlyVIA software Version 2.9.1 (Olympus Life Science; Tokyo, Japan). Kodachromes and archival paper photographs were scanned using the Epson Perfection V700 Photo Scanner (Epson Australia Pty Ltd., North Ryde, Australia).

2.9. Statistical Analysis

Statistical analysis was performed using GraphPad Prism 8 (GraphPad Software, San Diego, CA, USA) and SPSS Version 28 (IBM Corp, Armonk, NY, USA). The Fisher exact test was used to analyse (i) the presence of BLinD vs. Sarks Group I/II; (ii) RPE detachment on paraffin sections vs. the presence of BLinD upon TEM; and (iii) the presence of a sub-RPE space on semithin resin sections vs. the presence of BLinD upon TEM. A two-group *t*-test was used to evaluate the mean age and the mean number of TEM and semithin sections analysed between Sarks Groups I and II. Ordinal regression was used to analyse (i) BLinD grade vs. Group I/II; (ii) BrM hyalinisation grade vs. Group I/II; (iii) BrM hyalinisation vs. BLinD grade; (iv) BrM hyalinisation vs. age; (v) RPE microscopic morphology vs. Group I/II; and (vi) RPE morphology vs. BrM hyalinisation.

3. Results

3.1. Cohort

A total of 10 Sarks Group I (mean age 63.0 ± 8.3 years) and 16 Group II eyes (mean age 74.2 ± 7.3 years) (Figure 1) met the inclusion criteria summarised in Table 1. Group I eyes were significantly younger (p = 0.0014, 95% CI 4.8–17.6), with a trend towards better visual acuity (p = 0.11, 95% CI −0.05–0.5), compared with Group II. The interval between death and tissue fixation ranged from 1 to 12 h. The mean time from the last clinical review and patient death was 12.6 months in Group I and 18.1 months in Group II. There was no statistical difference in the number of semithin sections examined in Group I compared to Group II (7.5 ± 6.2 vs. 5.4 ± 3.8; p = 0.30, 95% CI −6.1–1.9) or in the number of TEM photographs reviewed per eye between the two groups (25.6 ± 20.4 vs. 19.0 ± 14.6; p = 0.34, 95% CI −20.7–7.53).

Table 1. Cohort characteristics. Ten normal Group I and 16 normal aged Group II eyes met the inclusion criteria. Compared with Group II eyes, the Group I eyes were significantly younger (p = 0.0014, 95% CI 4.8–17.6), with a trend towards better visual acuity (p = 0.11, 95% CI −0.05–0.5). The fundus was normal in all eyes at the last in vivo (clinical) examination, except for two eyes with non-specific pigment spots (noted as "vitelliform spots") seen in the context of a few small hard drusen.

Sarks Group [a]	Age (Years)	Sex	Post-Mortem Delay (Hours)	Visual Acuity [b] (LogMAR)	Follow-Up to Death Interval (Months)	Fundus Appearance Last Examination	Macular Paraffin Sections Reviewed	Macular Semithin Resin Sections Reviewed	Macular TEM Photographs Reviewed
Group I No macular BLamD									
1	73	M	Unknown	0	36	Normal	15	22	49
2	58	M	3	0	1	Normal	-	10	12
3	80	M	Unknown	0.18	36	Normal	-	4	6
4	55	M	Unknown	0	12	Normal	16	4	7
5	60	M	Unknown	0	5	Pigment spot	15	3	47
6	59	M	5	-	10	Normal	15	5	3
7	55	M	1	0	1	Normal	17	12	43
8	59	M	Unknown	0.18	10	Normal	20	10	55
9	69	M	Unknown	0	8	Normal	-	2	17
10	62	M	Unknown	0.18	7	Normal	15	3	17

Table 1. *Cont.*

Sarks Group [a]	Age (Years)	Sex	Post-Mortem Delay (Hours)	Visual Acuity [b] (LogMAR)	Follow-Up to Death Interval (Months)	Fundus Appearance Last Examination	Macular Paraffin Sections Reviewed	Macular Semithin Resin Sections Reviewed	Macular TEM Photographs Reviewed
Group II Patchy macular BLamD									
1	72	M	Unknown	−0.08	6	Normal	-	2	43
2	72	M	1.5 h	0	24	Normal	22	2	14
3	81	M	2 h	0.18	Unknown	Normal	15	6	55
4	74	M	12 h	0.18	2	Normal	-	8	11
5	74	M	12 h	0.8	2	Normal	-	7	2
6	88	M	Unknown	0.3	4	Normal	19	13	11
7	74	F	Unknown	0	9	Normal	-	9	16
8	74	F	Unknown	CF	9	Normal	-	1	12
9	72	M	Unknown	0.07	9	Normal	-	3	26
10	73	M	4.5 h	0.18	36	Normal	-	2	11
11	57	M	Unknown	0.3	31	Normal	-	12	30
12	66	M	Unknown	0.6	5	Normal	-	2	15
13	86	M	Unknown	0.18	5	Normal	18	2	17
14	77	M	11 h	0	64	Normal	-	8	2
15	77	M	11 h	0	64	Pigment spot	-	5	31
16	70	F	Unknown	0.18	1	Normal	15	5	8

[a] Histopathological grade based on the appearance of macular BLamD. [b] Corrected distance VA at last clinical visit. Abbreviations: VA—visual acuity; BLamD—basal laminar deposit; TEM—transmission electron microscopy.

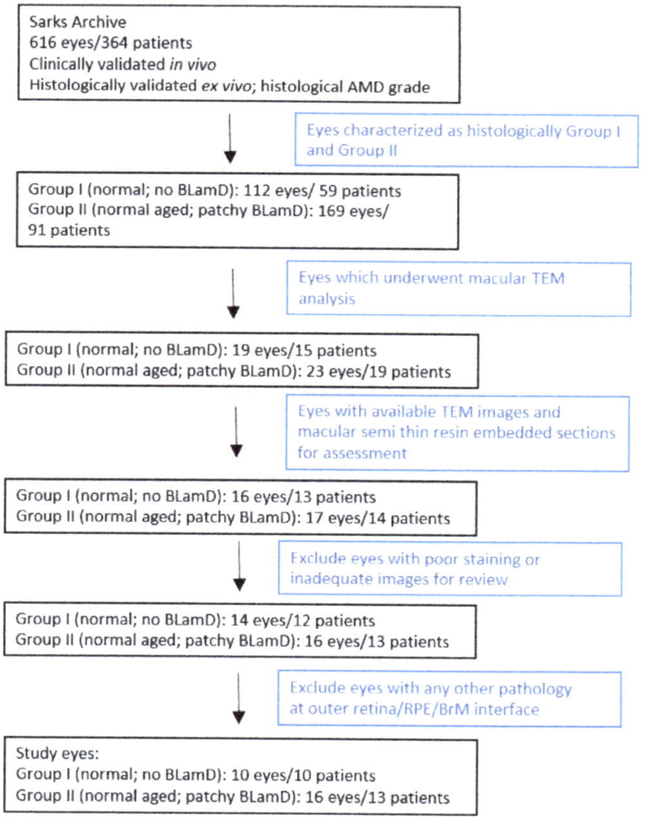

Figure 1. Study cohort: selection criteria. Abbreviations: BLamD—basal laminar deposit; TEM—transmission electron microscopy; RPE—retinal pigment epithelium; BrM—Bruch's membrane.

3.2. Basal Linear Deposit in Normal and Normal Aged Eyes

Electron-lucent vesicles were found in BrM in all study eyes. These were seen traversing through the RPE basement membrane and dispersed throughout all layers of BrM, from the inner to the outer collagenous zones. The vesicle size generally decreased with increasing distance from the RPE basement membrane as seen by TEM (Figures 2–6). A diffuse layer meeting our definition for BLinD was found in both normal (Group I) and normal aged (Group II) eyes (Table 2). Representative in vivo fundus photos and the corresponding macula paraffin, resin and TEM findings are shown in Figures 2 and 3. BLinD thickness grades are shown in Figures 4–6. BLinD was more frequently observed in Group II (10/16; 62.5%) compared with Group I (3/10; 30%) eyes. While this difference was not statistically significant (Fisher's exact test $p = 0.23$), the thickness of BLinD was greater in Group II (up to Grade 3) compared with Group I (up to Grade 2) (ordinal regression $p = 0.045$; 95% CI 0.04–3.4).

Table 2. BLinD in normal and normal aged eyes by ultrastructural analysis. BLinD was found in both normal Group I and normal aged Group II eyes. BrM hyalinisation was more advanced in Group II compared with Group I ($p = 0.013$; 95% CI 0.6–5.3), with a positive correlation between the degree of BrM hyalinisation and BLinD thickness ($p = 0.049$; 95% CI 0.05–2.69). The presence of BLinD in TEM photographs was not significantly associated with the RPE detachment seen in paraffin ($p > 0.99$) or resin sections ($p > 0.99$). There was no significant association between the RPE detachment seen in paraffin versus resin sections ($p = 0.12$).

Sarks Group [a]	Presence of BLinD [b]	BLinD Thickness (Grade) [b]	BrM Hyalinisation (Grade)	RPE Morphology	RPE Detachment in Paraffin Section	RPE Detachment in Semithin Resin Section
Group I No macular BLamD						
1	Present	1	2	Preserved	Diffuse	Focal
2	None	0	2	Preserved	-	None
3	Present	1	2	Preserved	-	Focal
4	Present	1	1	Foci of hypertrophy and hyperpigmentation	Diffuse	Focal
5	None	0	2	Preserved	Diffuse	Diffuse
6	None	0	2	Preserved	Diffuse	Focal
7	None	0	1	Preserved	Diffuse	None
8	None	0	1	Preserved	Diffuse	Diffuse
9	None	0	0	Preserved	-	Focal
10	None	0	1	Preserved	None	None
Group II Patchy macular BLamD						
1	Present	2	2	Preserved	-	None
2	None	0	2	Preserved	Focal	None
3	Present	2	2	Preserved	Diffuse	None
4	Present	1	2	Foci of hypo and hyperpigmentation	-	Focal
5	Present	1	2	Foci of hypo and hyperpigmentation	-	Focal
6	None	0	2	Preserved	Focal	None
7	Present	2	2	Abnormal	-	Focal
8	Present	2	2	Abnormal	-	Focal
9	Present	2	2	Preserved	-	None
10	None	0	2	Preserved	-	None
11	None	0	2	Preserved	-	None
12	None	0	1	Preserved	-	None
13	Present	1	3	Foci of hypo and hyperpigmentation	Diffuse	Diffuse
14	Present	2	3	Foci of hypopigmentation	-	Focal
15	Present	2	3	Foci of hypertrophy and thinning	-	None
16	None	0	3	Foci of hypertrophy	Focal	None

[a] Histopathological grade based on the appearance of macular BLamD. [b] Ultrastructural findings from TEM photographs of macular resin sections. - indicates that no paraffin sections were available for review. BLinD grades: 0 = none (less than the thickness of the RPE basement membrane; 0.3 µm); 1 = up to 3 × 0.3 µm; 2 = greater than 3 × 0.3 µm. Abbreviations: BLamD—basal laminar deposit; BLinD—basal linear deposit; BrM—Bruch's membrane; RPE—retinal pigment epithelium; TEM—transmission electron microscopy.

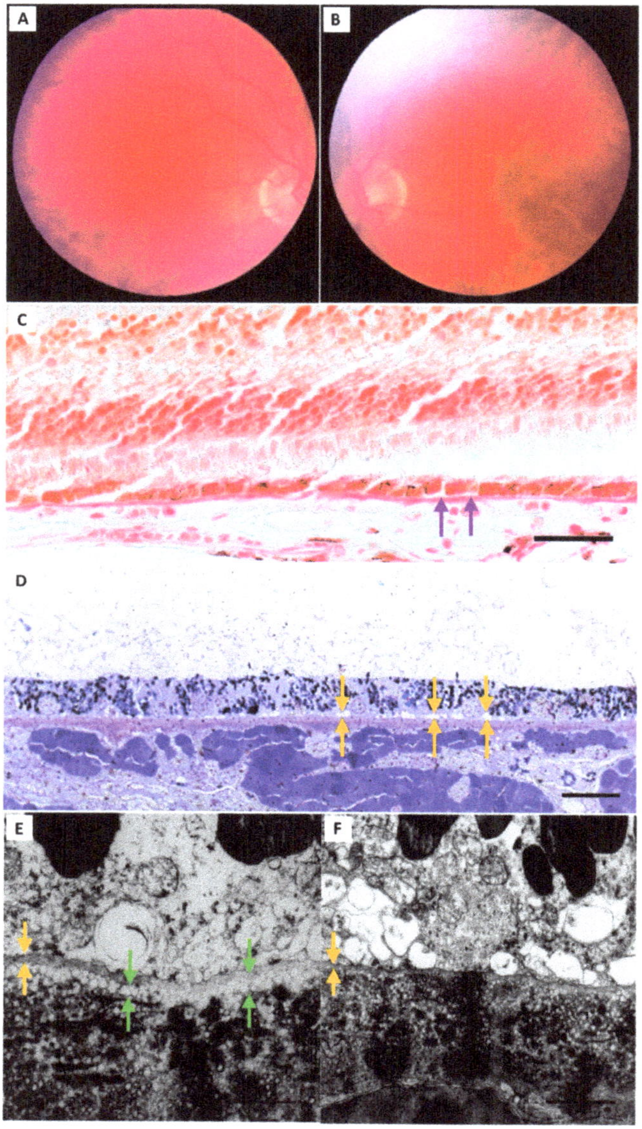

Figure 2. Study cohort: Group I (normal) eyes. epresentative Group I eye (55 year old male) with a normal bilateral fundus examination at the last clinical visit (**A**,**B**). Macular sections were examined under light (left and right eyes) and electron (right eye) microscopy. (**C**) Foci of RPE separation from BrM (purple arrows) are visible on the paraffin section of the macula. (**D**) In the semithin resin section, a small, unstained space is just visible between the base of the RPE and BrM (yellow arrows). (**E**) This space consists of a layer of vesicles when viewed by TEM (green arrows) and is external to the RPE basement membrane (yellow arrow). There is some variability in the thickness of this layer across different ultrastructural fields (**F**), seen here at 173,600× magnification. Scale bars: C = 20 µm; D = 20 µm; E = 1 µm; F = 1 µm. Paraffin section: picro-Mallory trichrome stain. Abbreviations: RPE—retinal pigment epithelium; BrM—Bruch's membrane; TEM—transmission electron microscopy.

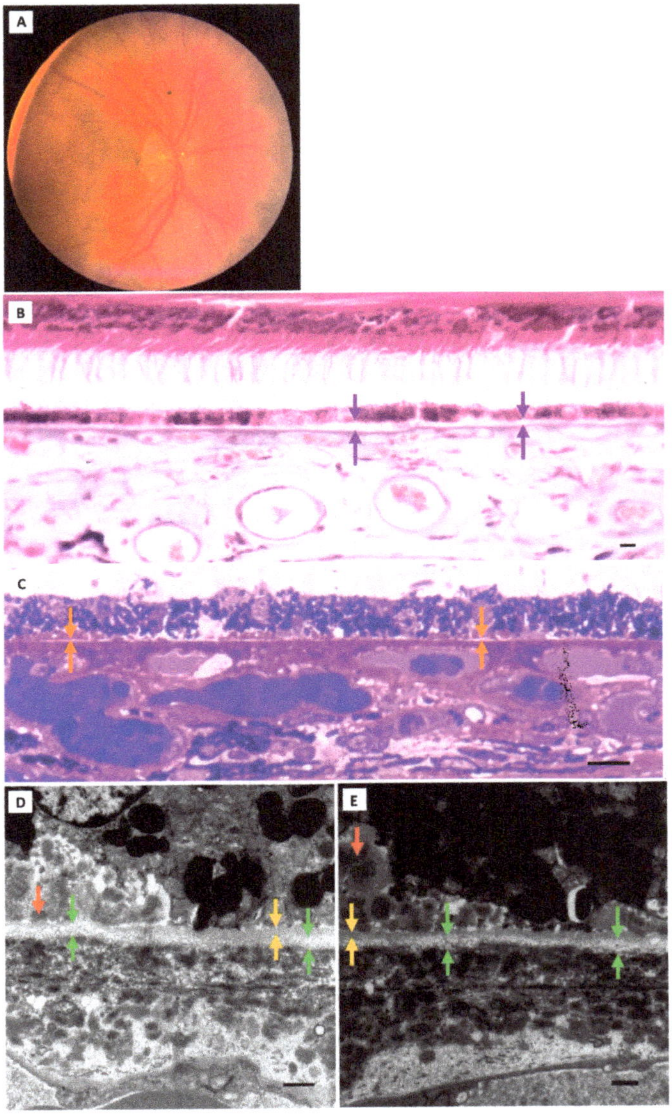

Figure 3. Study cohort: Group II (normal aged) eyes. (**A**) Representative Group II eye (85-year-old male). The fundus photo of the right eye at the last examination is shown. Macular sections were examined under light (left and right eyes) and electron (right eye) microscopy. (**B**) The macular paraffin section of the right eye shows diffuse RPE detachment (purple arrows) from BrM (Grade 3 hyalinisation). (**C**) In the semithin section, there are focal separations of the RPE (orange arrows) from the hyalinised BrM. Early-type BLamD is seen in thin patches (between asterisks). (**D**,**E**) In the TEM micrograph, BLinD (green arrows) is seen external to the RPE basement membrane (yellow arrows). Patchy BLamD (red arrows) is seen internal to the RPE basement membrane. Paraffin section scale bar = 15 µm; picro-Mallory trichrome stain. Resin section scale bar = 15 µm; toluidine blue stain. TEM scale bar: 1 µm. Abbreviations: RPE—retinal pigment epithelium; BLamD—basal laminar deposit; BLinD—basal linear deposit; TEM—transmission electron microscopy.

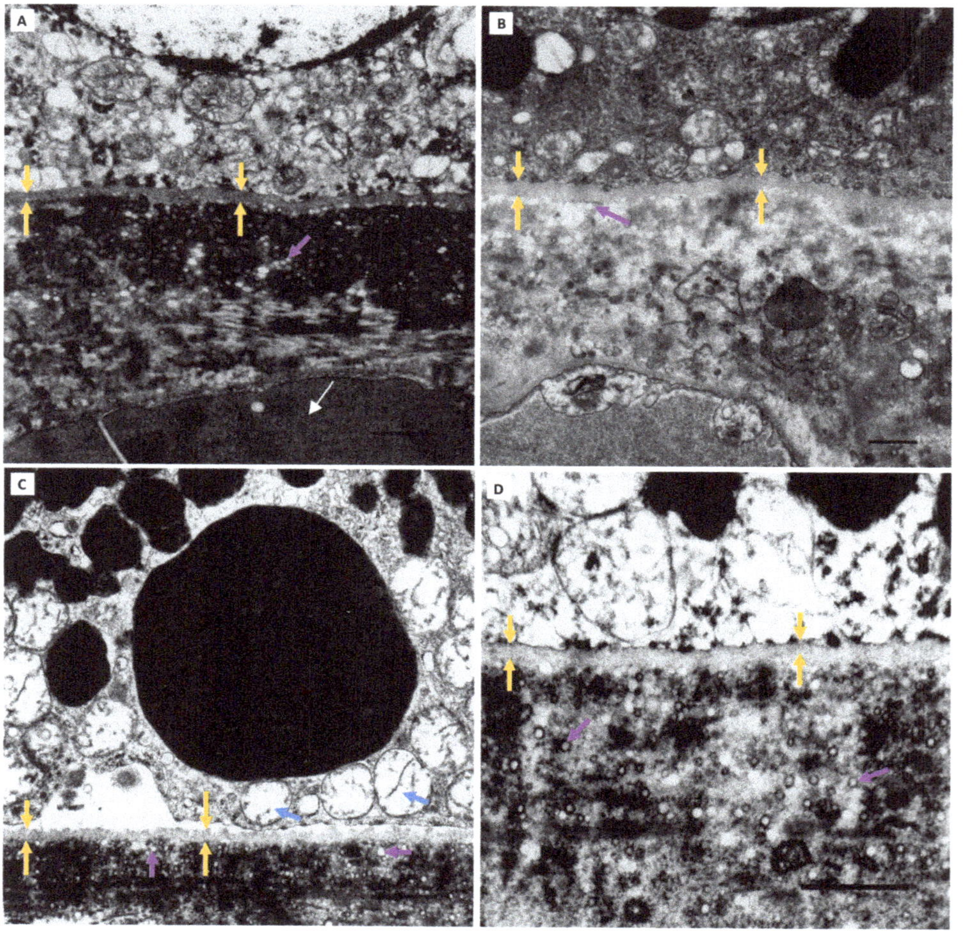

Figure 4. Grade 0 BLinD. Electron-lucent vesicles (purple arrows) external to the RPE basement membrane (yellow arrows) were present on the TEM micrographs in all study eyes, even those not meeting our definition for BLinD (a diffuse layer at least as thick as the RPE basement membrane). (**A**,**B**) TEM micrographs of two representative Group I (normal) eyes. Part of a choriocapillary red blood cell (white arrow) is captured. (**C**,**D**) Two representative Group II (normal aged) eyes with absent BLinD. Eyes without BLinD were almost twice as frequent in Group I (7/10; 70%) compared with Group II (6/16; 37.5%). The large, heterogenous, electron-dense structure next to mitochondria (blue arrow) in C likely represents melanolipofuscin. Scale bar: 1 µm. Abbreviations: RPE—retinal pigment epithelium; TEM—transmission electron microscopy; BLinD—basal linear deposit.

3.3. *Bruch's Membrane Hyalinisation, RPE Abnormalities and Basal Linear Deposit*

BrM was less hyalinised in Group I eyes (Grades 0 to 2) compared with Group II (Grades 1 to 3) (ordinal regression: $p = 0.013$; 95% CI 0.6–5.3). Increasing BrM hyalinisation was associated with increasing age across both groups (ordinal regression: $p < 0.08$, 95% CI 0.038–0.253) (Table 2). There was a positive correlation between BLinD thickness and the degree of BrM hyalinisation (ordinal regression $p = 0.049$; 95% CI 0.05–2.69). The morphology of the macular RPE was largely preserved and seen as a cuboidal monolayer in both groups, although mild abnormalities (focal decrease or increase in pigmentation, mild attenuation or hypertrophy) were more frequently observed in Group II ($p = 0.06$;

95% CI −0.89 to 4.484) (Table 2). Mild RPE abnormalities were positively correlated with both BrM hyalinisation (p = 0.044; 95% CI 0.61–4.319) and BLinD thickness (p = 0.022; 95% CI 0.188–2.422).

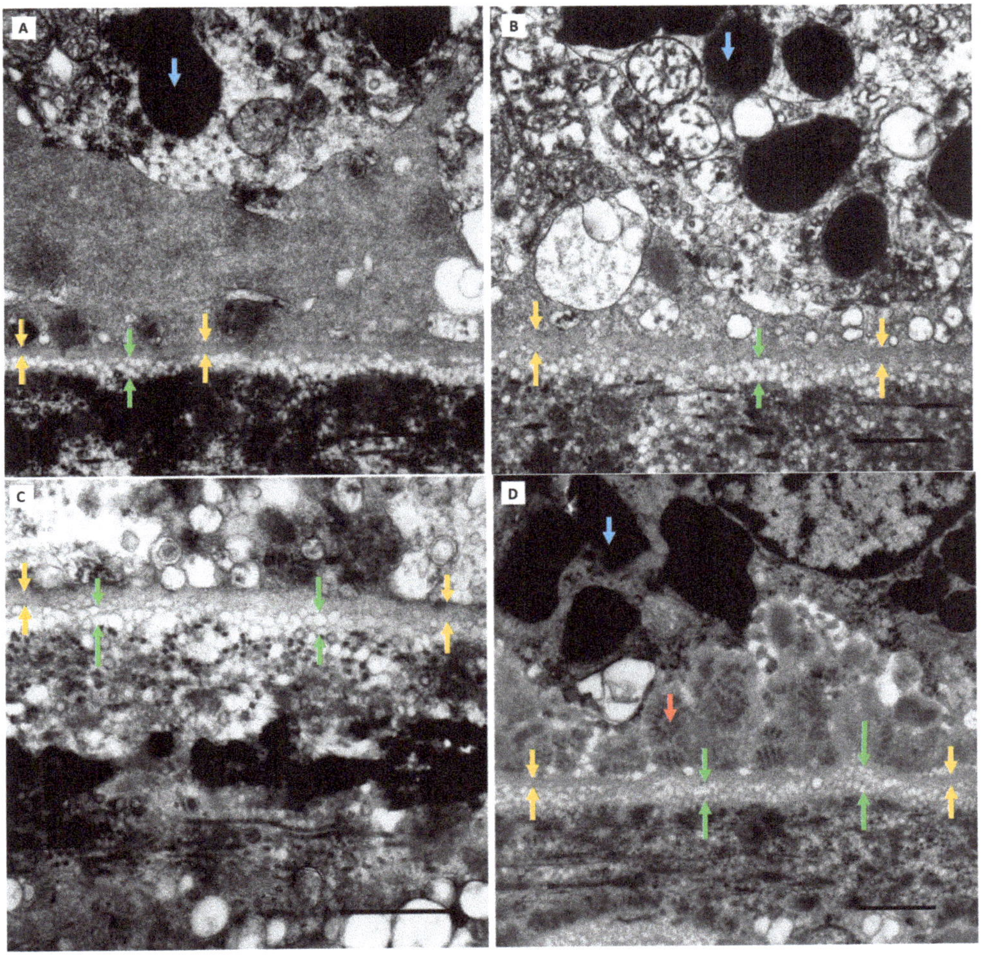

Figure 5. Grade 1 BLinD. Grade 1 BLinD (green arrows) was defined as up to 3 times the thickness of the RPE basement membrane (yellow arrows): 3 × 0.3 μm = approximately 0.9 μm was found in 2/10 Group I (normal) eyes and 3/16 Group II (normal aged) eyes. Macular TEM micrographs of Group I (**A**,**B**) and Group II eyes (**C**,**D**). Note the vesicles seen traversing the inner collagenous, elastic and outer collagenous layers of BrM, which become smaller and more dispersed with increasing distance from the RPE basement membrane. The larger vacuoles seen in (**C**,**D**) are within the cytoplasm of choriocapillary endothelial cells (best illustrated in (**D**)). Pigment granules (blue arrows) within the basal RPE cytoplasm are seen admixed with mitochondria. A patch of early-type BLamD, composed largely of long-spacing collagen (red arrow) is captured in (**D**). Scale bar: 1 μm. Abbreviations: BLinD—basal linear deposit; RPE—retinal pigment epithelium; TEM—transmission electron microscopy; BLamD—basal laminar deposit; BrM—Bruch's membrane.

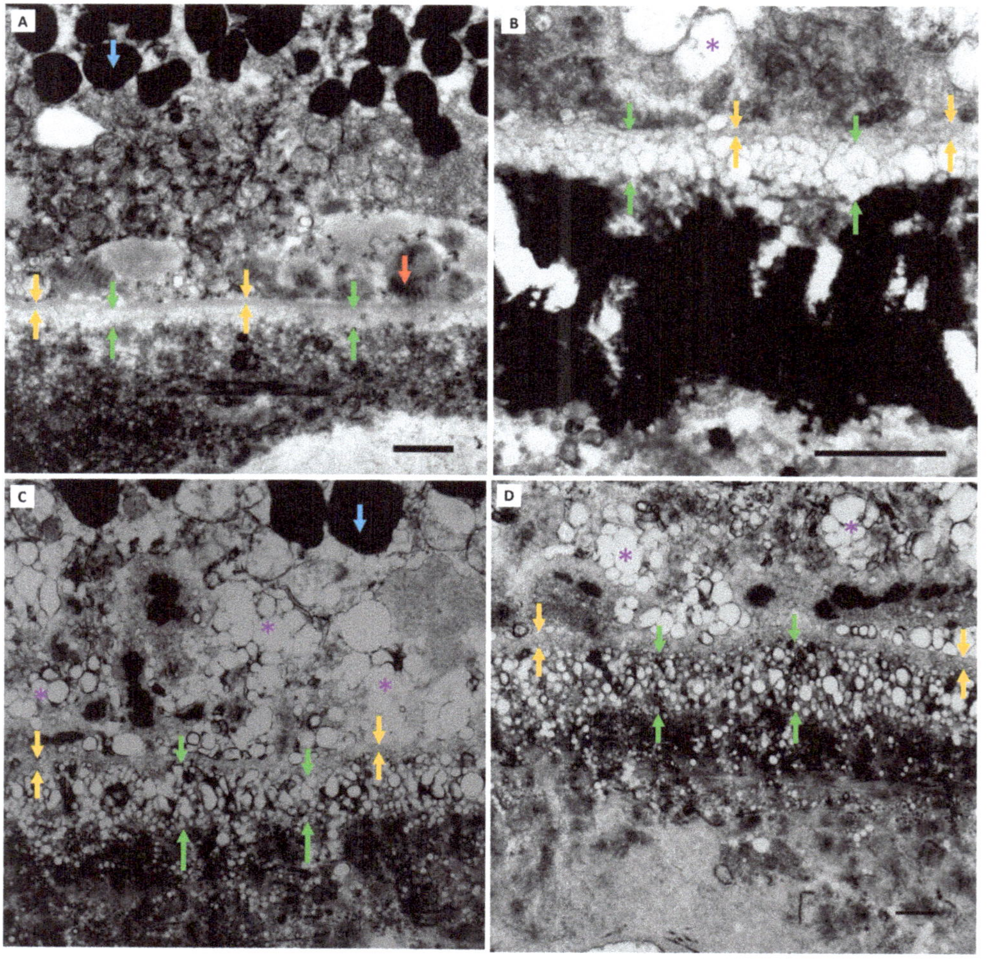

Figure 6. Grade 2 BLinD. Grade 2 BLinD (green arrows), defined as more than 3 times the thickness of the RPE basement membrane ($>3 \times 0.3$ μm ≥ 0.9 μm) (yellow arrows), was only seen in Group II (normal aged) eyes (7/16). Macular TEM micrographs of 4 representative Group II eyes are shown in (**A–D**). The blue arrows identify RPE cytoplasmic pigment granules. A patch of early-type BLamD (red arrow) is captured in (**A**). Again, electron-lucent vesicles are seen extending to the outer collagenous zone of BrM, decreasing in size and becoming sparser with increasing distance from the RPE basement membrane. Of note, larger lipid vesicles are seen internal to the RPE basement membrane, within the basal RPE cytoplasm (purple asterisk), best demonstrated in (**C**,**D**). TEM scale bar: 1 μm. Abbreviations: BLinD—basal linear deposit; RPE—retinal pigment epithelium; TEM—transmission electron microscopy; BLamD—basal laminar deposit; BrM—Bruch's membrane.

3.4. BLinD in AMD Eyes

Variations in BLinD thickness were observed between eyes in both Group I and II eyes and were also seen within the same eye across different TEM fields. To determine if this was also true for AMD eyes, we examined a representative clinically and histologically validated eye from Sarks Group III (early AMD) and Group IV (intermediate AMD). BLinD thickness also varied within both eyes (Figure 7). Group III and IV eyes also had a greater degree of

RPE detachment in semithin resin sections and more conspicuous RPE abnormalities by light microscopy.

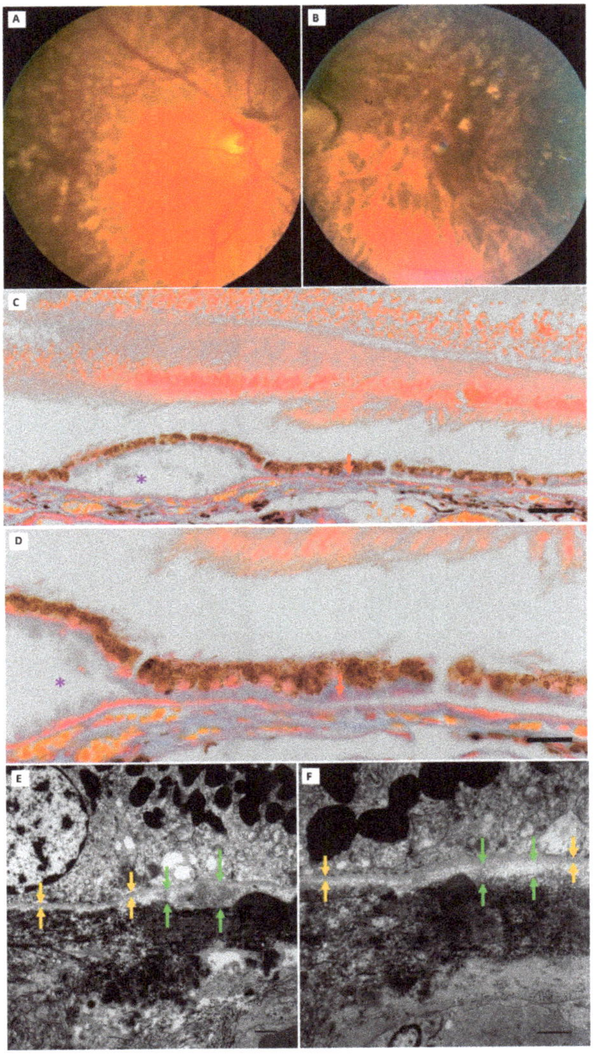

Figure 7. BLinD thickness in clinically and histologically validated AMD eyes. (**A**,**B**) A Sarks Group IV (intermediate AMD) eye (75-year-old male). Bilateral soft drusen and pigment changes at the last in vivo fundus examination. (**C**,**D**) Thick, continuous BLamD (red arrows) of both early (pale blue staining) and late (magenta inclusions) types is seen in the paraffin section of the left eye. Soft drusen appear as "optically empty" dome-shaped separations of both the RPE and BLamD from the hyalinised BrM (purple asterisk). RPE abnormalities are conspicuous, consisting of hypertrophy or attenuation and hyper- and hypopigmentation. Variability in BLinD thickness (green arrows) beneath the RPE-BM (yellow arrows) is seen in the right eye, shown here in two TEM fields (**E**,**F**) without soft drusen. Paraffin section scale: C = 50 µm, D = 20 µm. TEM scale bar: 1 µm. Abbreviations: BLinD—basal linear deposit; RPE—retinal pigment epithelium; TEM—transmission electron microscopy; BLamD—basal laminar deposit; BrM—Bruch's membrane.

3.5. RPE Detachment and BLinD

To determine if separation of the RPE from BrM on paraffin and resin sections could be used as a light microscopic marker of BLinD, we correlated this finding to the presence of BLinD upon TEM. RPE separation from BrM was more frequently seen in paraffin sections compared with resin sections (Table 2), and the degree of RPE separation was greater. Diffuse RPE separation was only seen in paraffin sections (Figure 8A). There was no significant association between the presence of BLinD by TEM and RPE separation in paraffin (Fisher's exact test $p > 0.99$) or resin ($p = 0.12$ for resin) sections. BLinD was observed in eyes with and without RPE separation in both paraffin and semithin sections (Figure 8). There was no association between the RPE separation observed in paraffin sections and the RPE separation observed in resin sections (Fisher's exact $p > 0.99$).

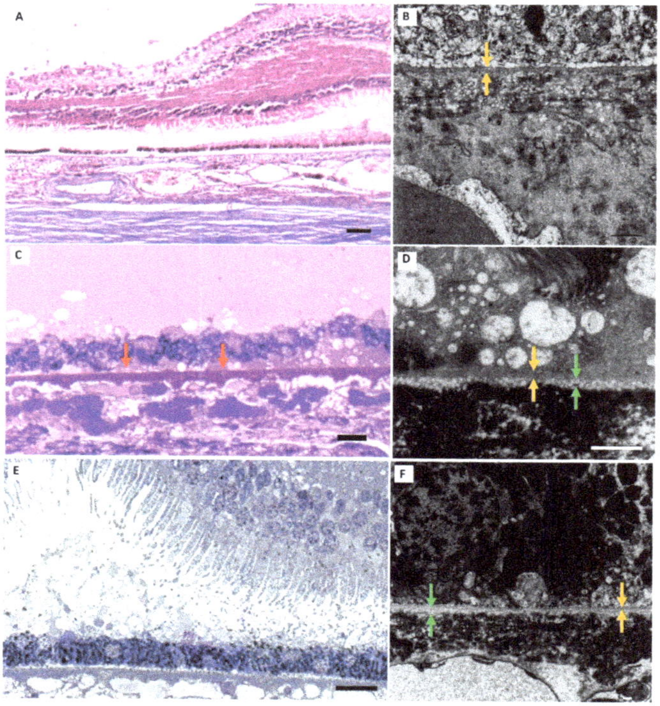

Figure 8. Separation of the RPE from BrM. RPE separation from BrM was not a reliable light microscopic marker for the presence of BLinD in this cohort of normal and normal aged eyes. A representative Group I eye with diffuse RPE detachment from BrM on paraffin section (**A**) and Grade 0 BLinD using TEM (**B**); note, instead, a layer of larger vesicles internal to the RPE basement membrane (yellow arrows). Areas of patchy BLamD (red arrows) and no RPE separation is seen in this macular semithin section (**C**) from a representative Group II eye with grade 1 BLinD (green arrows) by TEM (**D**). Diffuse separation of the RPE from BrM in the macular semithin section of a Group I eye (**E**) with grade 1 BLinD by TEM (**F**). TEM scale bar: 1 μm. Resin section scale bar: 15 μm. Paraffin section scale bar: 75 μm. Abbreviations: BLinD—basal linear deposit; RPE—retinal pigment epithelium; TEM—transmission electron microscopy; BLamD—basal laminar deposit; BrM—Bruch's membrane.

3.6. Diffuse Vesicle Layer Internal to the RPE Basement Membrane

In 3 of 26 normal and normal aged eyes, we observed a diffuse layer of electron-lucent vesicles internal to the RPE-BM by TEM (Figure 9). These vesicles were larger in size than those found within BLinD and often at least half the size of an RPE mitochondrion (at least 0.5 um). This layer has not been previously described in the published literature and was observed in two eyes with BLinD (n = 1 Group I; n = 1 Group II) and one eye without BLinD (Group I). There was no RPE detachment in the semithin sections for two of these eyes and focal detachment in one eye. Paraffin sections were available for one eye and showed diffuse RPE detachment. Identifying this layer prompted a review of all TEM micrographs of the study cohort. Similarly large, electron-lucent vesicles were seen in Group I and II eyes, irrespective of BLinD grade, but these did not form a continuous layer. There was, however, continuity between larger vesicles internal to the RPE basement membrane, smaller vesicles traversing the basement membrane, and BLinD external to the basement membrane (e.g., Figure 6C,D). Vesicles further extended into the elastin layer and outer collagenous zone of BrM, generally becoming smaller with increasing distance from the RPE.

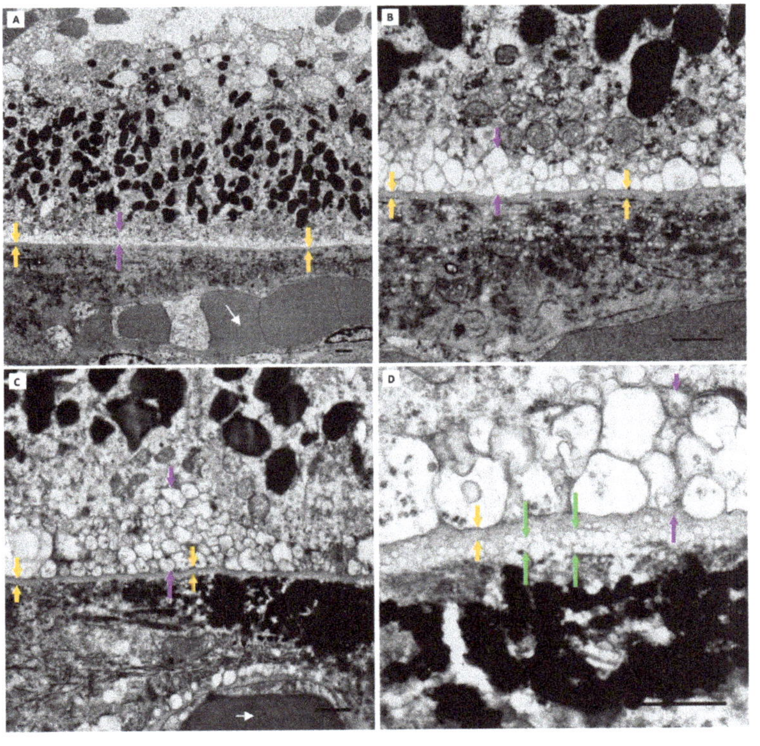

Figure 9. Diffuse layer of vesicles internal to the RPE basement membrane. A diffuse layer of larger, electron-lucent vesicles was seen in 3 of the 26 eyes in the normal and normal aged cohort. (**A**,**B**) A Group I eye with Grade 0 BLinD and a diffuse layer of large-vesicle deposition (purple arrows) internal to the RPE basement membrane (yellow arrows). (**C**,**D**). The same layer seen in another eye with Grade 1 BLinD (green arrows). Note the smaller electron-lucent vesicles traversing the RPE basement membrane (**D**) that extends into the inner collagenous zone through the elastin layer and into the outer collagenous zone of BrM (**B**), where some can be seen coalescing around the wall (**C**) of a choriocapillary. White arrows identify red blood cells in the choriocapillary lumen. TEM scale bar: 1 µm. Abbreviations: BLinD—basal linear deposit; RPE—retinal pigment epithelium; TEM—transmission electron microscopy.

4. Discussion

While the defining light microscopic lesion of AMD is the presence of continuous sub-macular BLamD, BLinD has, to date, been accepted as a co-occurring lesion observable by electron microscopy [3,4,19]. We found BLinD upon ultrastructural analysis of the RPE-BrM interface in a clinically and histologically validated cohort of adult human eyes *without* AMD. Because none of these eyes had continuous BLamD, our findings suggest that BLinD, when strictly defined, is likely an age-related lesion that precedes the onset of early AMD.

The use of a grading scale for BLinD thickness revealed an association with age, BrM hyalinisation and microscopic RPE abnormalities in this cohort of normal and normal aged eyes. This grading may be helpful in future studies to semi-quantitatively assess if age-related changes in BrM lipid content [6] is attributable to BLinD and whether BLinD thickness corresponds to AMD histological grade. BLinD was first described by Sarks as "an unbroken layer of vesicular membranous debris" external to the RPE basement membrane upon electron microscopic examination [5]. The same study defined undulations within this layer as soft drusen, and this was confirmed by correlation with soft drusen found through in vivo fundoscopy. The first published use of the term "BLinD" to describe this material appeared in 1993 and was defined as "vesicular material present throughout BrM", with each vesicle measuring "up to 120 nm" in diameter [13]. Our grading scale for BLinD is in accord with these original definitions and extends their utility by providing a semi-quantitative estimate. It may be helpful to clarify that the term "pre-BLinD", defined by Chen et al. [19] as a uniform, non-undulating layer ranging from 0.6–1.1 μm in thickness, is equivalent to BLinD Grades 1 to 2 in our study.

Our finding that BLinD thickness is correlated with both age and BrM hyalinisation also agrees with published observations. With ageing, there is a change in BrM matrix composition [20], reflected histologically by progressive degrees of hyalinisation [2,11]. Age-related BrM matrix changes are known to impede bidirectional transport between the RPE and photoreceptors [21–23]. These changes slow the transit of macromolecules and their carriers, some of which may manifest as the accumulations of debris within BrM.

In this study, the term "electron-lucent vesicle" is used purely as an ultrastructural descriptor of BLinD composition. In the general biological literature, a "vesicle" is defined as a sac bound by a selectively permeable, bilayered lipid membrane [24]. Extracellular vesicles facilitate intercellular communication and transport a wide array of biomolecules between cells, including proteins, nucleic acids, and lipids. The commonest extracellular vesicles observed in tissue are exosomes (30–100 nm) and microvesicles (100–1000 nm) [25]. While exosomes are derived from the endosomal pathway and microvesicles by directly budding from a cell's surface, both pathways are involved in physiological and pathological processes. Importantly, the cargo of both types of extracellular vesicles can be rich in lipids [26,27].

Several observations have been used to infer that BLinD is comprised of solid lipoprotein "particles" rather than vesicles. These include (i) the presence of esterified (bound) cholesterol in macular BrM [27], "basal deposits" and "drusen" [7]; (ii) the increased electron density of some BLinD constituents seen using lipid-preserving (OTAP) electron microscopy processing [8,28]; (iii) the presence of ApoB and ApoE (lipoproteins) in "basal deposits" and "drusen" [7]; and (iv) the appearance of spherical structures within BLinD by quick-freeze deep-etch scanning electron microscopy [29]. This biogenesis framework derives from an extensive range of published literature on the pathology of atheromatous plaques [30], which may be a poor fit to describe senescence-associated changes in bidirectional transport between RPE and the choriocapillaris. In atheroma pathogenesis, blood-derived lipoproteins are forced into an extracellular compartment (the vascular intima) under high arterial blood pressure, made possible once the barrier function of the endothelial monolayer is damaged [31]. This context shares few similarities with the physiological lipid transport that occurs between the RPE (neuroepithelium) and the choriocapillaris (low pressure, fenestrated capillary network) across a specialised extracellular matrix (BrM) within an immune-privileged intraocular microenvironment.

Lipoproteins act as vehicles for the transport of hydrophobic lipids within the aqueous environment of circulating blood; they are not a component of the normal extracellular matrix. Cell-to-cell transport of lipids, including esterified cholesterol and lipoproteins, occurs largely via extracellular vesicles [32,33]. Since BLinD can be found in normal eyes without AMD, its accumulation likely represents a physiological and dynamic process that increases with age and BrM hyalinisation.

Unless lipid transport between the RPE and the choriocapillaris can be uniquely established to occur via the release of free lipoproteins, it is likely that the cholesterol and lipoproteins observed within BrM and BLinD exist as the cargo of extracellular vesicles. This conceptual framework accommodates the key ultrastructural observations of BLinD. The electron-lucent vesicles in BLinD range from 50–200 nm in our study, which accords with previous observations [13]. Thus, they fall more within the range of exosomes and microvesicles (30–1000 nm) rather than lipoproteins (7–90 nm) [25,34]. More critically, BLinD vesicles are highly variable in both shape and size, whereas lipoproteins are uniformly shaped and sized [34]. Using the OTAP method, the most consistent finding is the electron-dense, lipid-rich outer membranes of BLinD structures [8], although there is insufficient evidence to determine if these are monolayer-like lipoproteins [8] or bilayer-like extracellular vesicles [3]. More importantly, OTAP reveals BLinD structures with a range of electron densities, from very dense to entirely lucent, suggesting a highly variable lipid content. This conflicts with findings expected for lipoproteins, which have a consistently high and uniform lipid content. The significance of the larger electron-lucent vesicles we found internal to the RPE basement membrane remains uncertain. However, the basolateral docking of vesicles prior to transport is biologically more plausible than attempting to fit this observation into the atheroma pathogenesis conceptual framework.

Limitations of this study include the unknown and long postmortem time to fixation in some eyes, which may have led to reduced tissue preservation. Furthermore, variation in fixation techniques (glutaraldehyde and formalin fixation) between paraffin and resin sections may have impacted the degree of RPE detachment observed and limited direct comparability. Additionally, thickness measurements may have been impacted by the angle at which the tissues were sectioned.

While our study is morphological, we contend that the science of BLinD biogenesis is far from settled, and that lipid transport mechanisms between the RPE and the choriocapillaris deserve further investigation. The point at which BLinD develops into soft drusen indicates the biological disease threshold for AMD. Evidence to date suggests that this threshold occurs when there is continuous macular BLamD [3]. Our data supports the use of BLinD grading to complement the AMD grading based on BLamD, serving to improve histopathological validation in study cohorts.

Author Contributions: Conceptualization, M.L., S.C., C.A. and V.P.; methodology, M.L., S.C., C.A., V.P. and A.L.T.; software, S.C., V.P. and J.A.; validation, M.C.M., S.C. and A.L.T.; formal analysis, A.L.T. and S.C.; investigation, A.L.T., S.C. and V.P.; resources, S.C., V.P. and J.A.; writing—original draft preparation, A.L.T., S.C. and M.C.M.; writing—review and editing, J.A., M.L., C.A. and V.P. supervision, M.C.M. and S.C.; project administration, V.P. All authors have read and agreed to the published version of the manuscript.

Funding: Funding was received from the Sarks Foundation (S.C.) and from Shirley and John Sarks via the Curran Foundation (V.P., M.L. and C.A.).

Institutional Review Board Statement: The study was conducted in accordance with the Declaration of Helsinki. The study protocol was approved by the St Vincent's Hospital Human Research Ethics Committee (REF: 2021/ETH01147) on 7 July 2021 and was monitored by the St Vincent's Hospital Sydney Research Office.

Informed Consent Statement: Data for this study were collected from within the Sarks archive. This archive consists of a cohort of eyes from prospectively consented patients obtained from 1967 to 1995.

Data Availability Statement: The original contributions presented in the study are included in the article; further inquiries can be directed to the corresponding author/s.

Acknowledgments: The authors acknowledge the lifetime work of Shirley and John Sarks. This study's clinically and histologically validated cohort would not be available without their decades-long dedication and commitment. We would like to acknowledge the greatly valued input of Christine A. Curcio in this manuscript. We acknowledge the technical assistance of Iveta Slapetova and Maria Kasherman (Katharina Gaus Light Microscopy Facility, UNSW, Sydney) for digital slide scanning advice.

Conflicts of Interest: The authors report no conflicts of interest in this work.

References

1. Age-Related Eye Disease Study Research Group. The Age-Related Eye Disease Study system for classifying age-related macular degeneration from stereoscopic color fundus photographs: The Age-Related Eye Disease Study Report Number 6. *Am. J. Ophthalmol.* **2001**, *132*, 668–681. [CrossRef] [PubMed]
2. Sarks, S.H. Ageing and degeneration in the macular region: A clinico-pathological study. *Br. J. Ophthalmol.* **1976**, *60*, 324–341. [CrossRef] [PubMed]
3. Sarks, S.; Cherepanoff, S.; Killingsworth, M.; Sarks, J. Relationship of Basal Laminar Deposit and Membranous Debris to the Clinical Presentation of Early Age-Related Macular Degeneration. *Investig. Ophthalmol. Vis. Sci.* **2007**, *48*, 968–977. [CrossRef] [PubMed]
4. Curcio, C.A.; Millican, C.L. Basal linear deposit and large drusen are specific for early age-related maculopathy. *Arch. Ophthalmol.* **1999**, *117*, 329–339. [CrossRef] [PubMed]
5. Sarks, S.H. Council Lecture. Drusen and their relationship to senile macular degeneration. *Aust. J. Ophthalmol.* **1980**, *8*, 117–130. [CrossRef] [PubMed]
6. Pauleikhoff, D.; Harper, C.A.; Marshall, J.; Bird, A.C. Aging changes in Bruch's membrane. A histochemical and morphologic study. *Ophthalmology* **1990**, *97*, 171–178. [CrossRef] [PubMed]
7. Malek, G.; Li, C.M.; Guidry, C.; Medeiros, N.E.; Curcio, C.A. Apolipoprotein B in cholesterol-containing drusen and basal deposits of human eyes with age-related maculopathy. *Am. J. Pathol.* **2003**, *162*, 413–425. [CrossRef] [PubMed]
8. Curcio, C.A.; Presley, J.B.; Millican, C.L.; Medeiros, N.E. Basal deposits and drusen in eyes with age-related maculopathy: Evidence for solid lipid particles. *Exp. Eye Res.* **2005**, *80*, 761–775. [CrossRef]
9. Sarks, S.H.; Van Driel, D.; Maxwell, L.; Killingsworth, M. Softening of drusen and subretinal neovascularization. *Trans. Ophthalmol. Soc. U. K.* **1980**, *100*, 414–422.
10. Penfold, P.L.; Killingsworth, M.C.; Sarks, S.H. Senile macular degeneration. The involvement of giant cells in atrophy of the retinal pigment epithelium. *Investig. Ophthalmol. Vis. Sci.* **1986**, *27*, 364–371.
11. van der Schaft, T.L.; Mooy, C.M.; de Bruijn, W.C.; Oron, F.G.; Mulder, P.G.H.; de Jong, P.T.V.M. Histologic Features of the Early Stages of Age-related Macular Degeneration: A Statistical Analysis. *Ophthalmology* **1992**, *99*, 278–286. [CrossRef] [PubMed]
12. Marshall, G.E.; Konstas, A.G.; Reid, G.G.; Edwards, J.G.; Lee, W.R. Type IV collagen and laminin in Bruch's membrane and basal linear deposit in the human macula. *Br. J. Ophthalmol.* **1992**, *76*, 607–614. [CrossRef] [PubMed]
13. Green, W.R.; Enger, C. Age-related Macular Degeneration Histopathologic Studies: The 1992 Lorenz E. Zimmerman Lecture. *Ophthalmology* **1993**, *100*, 1519–1535. [CrossRef]
14. Sarks, J.P.; Sarks, S.H.; Killingsworth, M.C. Evolution of soft drusen in age-related macular degeneration. *Eye* **1994**, *8 Pt 3*, 269–283. [CrossRef]
15. Guyer, D.R.; Schachat, A.P.; Green, W.R. Chapter 3—The Choroid: Structural Considerations. In *Retina*, 4th ed.; Ryan, S.J., Hinton, D.R., Schachat, A.P., Wilkinson, C.P., Eds.; Mosby: Edinburgh, UK, 2006; pp. 33–42.
16. Westerman, M.P.; Pierce, L.E.; Jensen, W.N. A direct method for the quantitative measurement of red cell dimensions. *J. Lab. Clin. Med.* **1961**, *57*, 819–824.
17. Thumann, G.; Dou, G.; Wang, Y.; Hinton, D.R. Chapter 16—Cell Biology of the Retinal Pigment Epithelium. In *Retina*, 5th ed.; Ryan, S.J., Sadda, S.R., Hinton, D.R., Schachat, A.P., Sadda, S.R., Wilkinson, C.P., Wiedemann, P., Schachat, A.P., Eds.; W.B. Saunders: London, UK, 2013; pp. 401–414.
18. Forrester, J.V.; Dick, A.D.; McMenamin, P.G.; Roberts, F.; Pearlman, E. Chapter 1—Anatomy of the eye and orbit. In *The Eye*, 4th ed.; Forrester, J.V., Dick, A.D., McMenamin, P.G., Roberts, F., Pearlman, E., Eds.; W.B. Saunders: Edinburgh, UK, 2016; pp. 1–102.e2.
19. Chen, L.; Messinger, J.D.; Kar, D.; Duncan, J.L.; Curcio, C.A. Biometrics, Impact, and Significance of Basal Linear Deposit and Subretinal Drusenoid Deposit in Age-Related Macular Degeneration. *Investig. Ophthalmol. Vis. Sci.* **2021**, *62*, 33. [CrossRef] [PubMed]
20. Newsome, D.A.; Huh, W.; Green, W.R. Bruch's membrane age-related changes vary by region. *Curr. Eye Res.* **1987**, *6*, 1211–1221. [CrossRef]
21. Moore, D.J.; Clover, G.M. The Effect of Age on the Macromolecular Permeability of Human Bruch's Membrane. *Investig. Ophthalmol. Vis. Sci.* **2001**, *42*, 2970–2975.
22. Moore, D.J.; Hussain, A.A.; Marshall, J. Age-related variation in the hydraulic conductivity of Bruch's membrane. *Investig. Ophthalmol. Vis. Sci.* **1995**, *36*, 1290–1297.

23. Starita, C.; Hussain, A.A.; Pagliarini, S.; Marshall, J. Hydrodynamics of ageing Bruch's membrane: Implications for macular disease. *Exp. Eye Res.* **1996**, *62*. 565–572. [CrossRef]
24. Morshed, A.; Karawdeniya, B.I.; Bandara, Y.; Kim, M.J.; Dutta, P. Mechanical characterization of vesicles and cells: A review. *Electrophoresis* **2020**, *41*, 449–470. [CrossRef] [PubMed]
25. Colombo, M.; Raposo, G.; Théry, C. Biogenesis, secretion, and intercellular interactions of exosomes and other extracellular vesicles. *Annu. Rev. Cell Dev. Biol.* **2014**, *30*, 255–289. [CrossRef] [PubMed]
26. Skotland, T.; Sagini, K.; Sandvig, K.; Llorente, A. An emerging focus on lipids in extracellular vesicles. *Adv. Drug Deliv. Rev.* **2020**, *159*, 308–321. [CrossRef] [PubMed]
27. Fyfe, J.; Casari, I.; Manfredi, M.; Falasca, M. Role of lipid signalling in extracellular vesicles-mediated cell-to-cell communication. *Cytokine Growth Factor Rev.* **2023**, *73*, 20–26. [CrossRef]
28. Curcio, C.A.; Millican, C.L.; Bailey, T.; Kruth, H.S. Accumulation of cholesterol with age in human Bruch's membrane. *Investig. Ophthalmol. Vis. Sci.* **2001**, *42*, 265–274.
29. Ruberti, J.W.; Curcio, C.A.; Millican, C.L.; Menco, B.P.; Huang, J.D.; Johnson, M. Quick-freeze/deep-etch visualization of age-related lipid accumulation in Bruch's membrane. *Investig. Ophthalmol. Vis. Sci.* **2003**, *44*, 1753–1759. [CrossRef]
30. Curcio, C.A.; Johnson, M.; Rudolf, M.; Huang, J.D. The oil spill in ageing Bruch membrane. *Br. J. Ophthalmol.* **2011**, *95*, 1638–1645. [CrossRef] [PubMed]
31. Rafieian-Kopaei, M.; Setorki, M.; Doudi, M.; Baradaran, A.; Nasri, H. Atherosclerosis: Process, indicators, risk factors and new hopes. *Int. J. Prev. Med.* **2014**, *5*, 927–946. [PubMed]
32. Pfrieger, F.W.; Vitale, N. Cholesterol and the journey of extracellular vesicles. *J. Lipid Res.* **2018**, *59*, 2255–2261. [CrossRef]
33. Reiss, A.B.; Vernice, N.A.; Siegart, N.M.; De Leon, J.; Kasselman, L.J. Exosomes in Cholesterol Metabolism and Atherosclerosis. *Cardiovasc. Hematol. Disord. Drug Targets* **2017**, *17*, 185–194. [CrossRef]
34. German, J.B.; Smilowitz, J.T.; Zivkovic, A.M. Lipoproteins: When size really matters. *Curr. Opin. Colloid Interface Sci.* **2006**, *11*, 171–183. [CrossRef] [PubMed]

Journal of
Clinical Medicine

MDPI

Article

Nationwide Screening Practices for Tamoxifen Retinal Toxicity in South Korea: A Population-Based Cohort Study

Seong Joon Ahn [1,*], Jiyeong Kim [2] and Hyeon Yoon Kwon [1]

[1] Department of Ophthalmology, Hanyang University Hospital, Hanyang University College of Medicine, 222-1 Wangsipli-ro, Seongdong-gu, Seoul 04763, Republic of Korea
[2] Department of Pre-Medicine, College of Medicine, and Biostatistics Lab, Medical Research Collaborating Center (MRCC), Hanyang University, Seoul 04763, Republic of Korea
* Correspondence: ahnsj81@gmail.com; Tel.: +82-2-2290-8574; Fax: +82-2-2291-8517

Abstract: (1) Background/Objectives: To investigate the nationwide screening practices and trends in tamoxifen retinal toxicity (tamoxifen retinopathy) in South Korea using national health insurance claims data. **(2) Methods:** A total of 43,848 patients who started tamoxifen therapy between 2015 and 2020 and had no prior ophthalmic diseases or other conditions requiring screening for retinopathy were included. The annual numbers of tamoxifen users and new initiators of tamoxifen therapy were assessed. The screening examinations were separated into baseline (first ophthalmic examination after tamoxifen administration) and subsequent monitoring examinations. The timing and modalities for the baseline and subsequent monitoring examinations performed between 2015 and 2021 were assessed in tamoxifen users. **(3) Results:** The annual number of tamoxifen users increased over the study period from 54,056 in 2015 to 81,720 in 2021. The number of patients who underwent ophthalmic examination after tamoxifen administration was 8961 (20.4%). Baseline screening was performed in 6.5% of patients within 1 year of use, and subsequent monitoring was performed in 27.8% of patients who underwent baseline screening. Funduscopy or fundus photography was performed most commonly for baseline screening and subsequent monitoring (99.0% and 98.6%, respectively), while optical coherence tomography was performed only in 21.9% and 29.6% of baseline and monitoring examinations, respectively. The average number of monitoring examinations per year was 0.68 ± 0.45. Although the annual percentage of patients receiving a baseline examination within 1 year gradually increased over time, the percentage of those with subsequent monitoring performed within 1 year was similar over the study period. **(4) Conclusions:** Our finding, appropriate screening in a small proportion of patients receiving tamoxifen, suggests the need to promote awareness among healthcare professionals and develop a standardized approach for screening for tamoxifen retinopathy.

Keywords: drug usage; retinal toxicity; screening practices; tamoxifen

1. Introduction

Tamoxifen, a selective estrogen receptor (ER) modulator, is widely used to treat and prevent hormone-receptor-positive breast cancer [1,2]. It has proven effective in reducing the risk of cancer recurrence and improving survival rates in women with ER-positive breast tumors [3,4]. However, long-term use of tamoxifen has been associated with ocular side effects, including tamoxifen retinopathy, a condition that affects the retina and potentially leads to vision loss [1,5,6].

Tamoxifen retinal toxicity, namely, tamoxifen retinopathy, typically manifests as a bilateral symmetrical condition, although asymmetrical involvement can also occur. The clinical features of tamoxifen retinopathy vary from mild to severe. The common signs of tamoxifen retinopathy include crystalline deposits within the macula, known as refractile bodies or tamoxifen crystals [1]. These deposits are often observed in the inner retinal layers and can be visualized by fundus examination. As the condition progresses, other characteristic findings may emerge, such as retinal pigment epithelial changes including granularity, mottling, and pigment clumping. Pseudocystic macular changes and edema may develop, leading to visual disturbances [2]. In advanced stages of tamoxifen retinopathy, retinal atrophy and optic disc pallor may be observed [7].

Accordingly, the timely detection of tamoxifen retinopathy is crucial for implementing appropriate interventions to prevent irreversible structural and functional (vision) loss [1]. Unfortunately, recommendations have not yet been provided by expert panels or organizations, nor has there been a consensus on the screening frequency and modalities for tamoxifen retinopathy. Nationwide practice patterns for tamoxifen retinopathy screening have not yet been reported.

This study intended to investigate practice patterns for screening for tamoxifen retinopathy in Korean population. We aimed to explore the timing and diagnostic modalities employed in screening for retinopathy and highlight the challenges and limitations of real-world practice in Korea.

2. Materials and Methods

2.1. Study Population

The participants in this cohort study were identified using the Health Insurance Review and Assessment database, which holds comprehensive health claims data for approximately 50 million individuals in South Korea. This database includes detailed records of medication prescriptions, visit dates, and demographic information, along with diagnoses categorized according to the Korean Standard Classification of Diseases, 8th Revision, with adaptations based on the International Statistical Classification of Diseases and Related Health Problems, Tenth Revision (ICD-10). From the database, we identified tamoxifen users who were treated with tamoxifen between 1 January 2012 and 31 December 2021. Patients who had used tamoxifen before 1 January 2015 were excluded to obtain the population who started the therapy between 2015 and 2021 (and thus their treatment duration could be accurately assessed within the study period).

Additionally, individuals who had undergone ophthalmic examinations, including fundus photography or optical coherence tomography (OCT), for any preexisting ophthalmic disease (ICD-10 codes H00-H59) before the initiation of tamoxifen treatment or those with diabetes mellitus or common ophthalmic diseases were excluded to eliminate visits scheduled for monitoring preexisting or common eye diseases or diabetic retinopathy. Further details of the inclusion and exclusion criteria, as well as the number of patients, are presented in Figure 1.

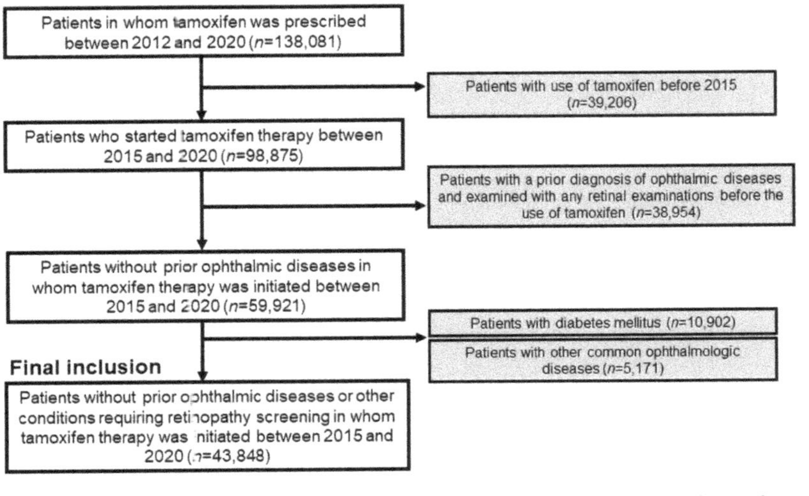

Figure 1. A flowchart of the study population and inclusion/exclusion criteria in this study.

The study was approved by the Institutional Review Board of Hanyang University Hospital (IRB file no. 2023-01-003) and conducted in accordance with the principles of the Declaration of Helsinki. The need for informed consent was waived by the Institutional Review Board of Hanyang University Hospital because of the retrospective nature of the study and the use of deidentified data.

2.2. Definitions and Evaluations

Several definitions are used in this study. Baseline examination was defined as the first ophthalmic examination performed after the initiation of tamoxifen therapy as the initial assessment of retinal toxicity associated with tamoxifen use. Subsequent monitoring was defined as examinations performed after baseline examination [8].

Several parameters and outcome measures were evaluated as follows. First, we evaluated the annual number of tamoxifen users from 2015 to 2021. This provided the trends and changes in total and new tamoxifen users. Second, the timing of the examinations, baseline or subsequent monitoring, was assessed. Together with the interval between the start date of tamoxifen use and baseline examination, and that between baseline and subsequent monitoring examinations, we examined the frequency of patients who underwent baseline screening within 1 year of initiating tamoxifen therapy, as well as the percentage of patients receiving subsequent monitoring within 6 months and 1 year from the time of baseline screening. The modalities used for baseline screening and subsequent monitoring examinations were also documented. We specifically recorded the use of OCT, funduscopy/fundus photography, automated visual field (VF), fundus autofluorescence (FAF), and fluorescein angiography (FA) for both baseline and monitoring examinations to obtain information on the preferred diagnostic techniques for screening for tamoxifen-induced retinal toxicity. Finally, the number of monitoring examinations per year was calculated to assess the frequency at which patients underwent subsequent monitoring examinations.

2.3. Data Analysis

This study employed descriptive statistics to summarize and present the findings. Categorical variables are presented as frequencies and percentages, while continuous variables are reported as mean (standard deviation) or median (interquartile range) values. Fisher's exact or Chi-square tests were used to compare categorical variables between groups. All p-values are based on two-sided tests, and statistical significance was considered at $p < 0.05$. Statistical analyses were conducted using SAS Enterprise Guide version 7.1 (SAS Institute, Cary, NC, USA).

3. Results

3.1. Population of Tamoxifen Users and Trends over Time

In our study, we identified 43,848 tamoxifen users without prior ophthalmic diseases or conditions requiring retinopathy screening, of whom 88.6% were female. The demographic and clinical characteristics of tamoxifen users included in this study are presented in Table 1. The mean age of the users was 45.0 ± 9.7 years. In terms of age groups, most users were 40–49 years old (54.0%), followed by 50–59 years old (18.0%). The indications for tamoxifen use varied, with breast cancer being the most common (69.9%), followed by ductal carcinoma in situ (17.7%) and gynecomastia (10.5%). The mean duration of tamoxifen use was 36.0 ± 21.8 months, and the mean daily dose was 20.0 ± 3.0 mg.

The annual trends in the number of overall tamoxifen users and initiators between 2015 and 2021 are presented in Table 2, and the proportion of users in the entire Korean population each year is also depicted in the table. In 2015, there were 54,056 patients using tamoxifen, accounting for 0.106% of the Korean population. The number of patients who initiated tamoxifen therapy that year was 14,065, representing 0.028% of the Korean population. Over the subsequent years, both the total number of tamoxifen users and the number of patients who initiated therapy gradually increased. By 2021, the total number of patients using tamoxifen reached 81,720, comprising 0.158% of the Korean population, while 18,012 patients initiated tamoxifen therapy, accounting for 0.035% of the population. These findings demonstrate an increasing trend in the numbers of tamoxifen users and initiators over the study period, indicating an increasing population at risk of tamoxifen-induced retinal toxicity in South Korea.

Table 1. Demographic and clinical information of the tamoxifen users included in this study.

Characteristics	Overall Users (n = 43,848)
Sex	
Male	5003 (11.4%)
Female	38,845 (88.6%)
Mean age (±SD), years	45.0 ± 9.7
<20	688 (1.6%)
20–29	1860 (4.2%)
30–39	6968 (15.9%)
40–49	23,667 (54.0%)
50–59	7903 (18.0%)
60–69	1945 (4.4%)
≥70	817 (1.9%)
Indication for tamoxifen use	
Breast cancer	30,629 (69.9%)
Ductal carcinoma in situ	7744 (17.7%)
Gynecomastia	4606 (10.5%)
Others	869 (2.0%)
Mean duration of tamoxifen use (±SD), months	36.0 ± 21.8
Less than 1 year	7858 (17.9%)
1–2 years	6287 (14.3%)
2–3 years	7857 (17.9%)
3–4 years	6849 (15.6%)
4–5 years	8715 (19.9%)
5 years or longer	6282 (14.3%)
Mean daily dose of tamoxifen (±SD), mg/day	20.0 ± 3.0
Less than 15 mg	1064 (2.4%)
15–20 mg	808 (1.8%)
20–25 mg	41,261 (94.1%)
25 mg or greater	715 (1.6%)

SD, standard deviation.

Table 2. Annual number of tamoxifen users and those who started tamoxifen therapy between 2015 and 2021.

Year	Total Number of Patients Using Tamoxifen (% among Entire Korean Population in Each Year †)	Annual Number of Patients Who Initiated Tamoxifen Therapy (% among Korean Population †)
2015	54,056 (0.106%)	14,065 (0.028%)
2016	59,426 (0.116%)	15,690 (0.031%)
2017	64,760 (0.126%)	16,689 (0.032%)
2018	69,957 (0.136%)	17,272 (0.033%)
2019	74,860 (0.145%)	17,990 (0.035%)
2020	77,943 (0.150%)	17,169 (0.033%)
2021	81,720 (0.158%)	18,012 (0.035%)

† Obtained by dividing the number of tamoxifen users by that of the entire Korean population in each year (from 51,014,947 in 2015 to 51,744,876 in 2021).

3.2. Performance, Timing, and Modalities of Baseline and Subsequent Monitoring Examinations

Only a small proportion (6.5%) of the study population underwent baseline screening within 1 year of initiating tamoxifen therapy (Table 3). The proportion of patients who underwent ophthalmic examination at any time after tamoxifen administration was 20.4%. Figure S1 shows the timing of baseline screening from the start date of tamoxifen treatment, showing a gradual decrease in percentages over time. Funduscopy/fundus photography was the most commonly used modality for baseline screening and was performed in 99.0% of cases. OCT was used in only 21.9% of patients who underwent baseline examinations. A small fraction of patients underwent automated VF (6.7%), FAF (2.8%), and FA (0.8%).

Table 3. Descriptive statistics of the timing and modalities used for the baseline examination (1st ophthalmic examination after tamoxifen use) and monitoring (subsequent follow-up screening) among all patients between 2015 and 2021.

Characteristics	Value
Timing	
No. of patients receiving any ophthalmic examination after tamoxifen use/No. of users (%)	8961/43,848 (20.4%)
No. of patients receiving ophthalmic examination within 1 year of tamoxifen use/No. of users (%)	2836/43,848 (6.5%)
No. of patients receiving any subsequent monitoring examination/No. of patients receiving baseline screening (%)	2492/8961 (27.8%)
No. of monitoring examinations per year after baseline ones, numbers/year	0.68 ± 0.45
Timing of the baseline examination since tamoxifen use, median (Q1–Q3), days	645 (280–1161)
Mean/median (Q1–Q3) interval between baseline examination and 1st monitoring exam, months	12.5 ± 14.2/7.1 (1.2–19.3)
Mean/median (Q1–Q3) interval of monitoring between 1st and 2nd monitoring exam, months	6.9 ± 8.7/3.4 (0.7–10.1)
Mean/median (Q1–Q3) interval of monitoring between 2nd and 3rd monitoring exam, months	5.8 ± 8.4/2.8 (0.6–7.1)
Modalities used	Baseline/Monitoring (%)
Funduscopy/fundus photography	8873 (99.0%)/2458 (98.6%)
Optical coherence tomography	1960 (21.9%)/738 (29.6%)
Automated visual fields	602 (6.7%)/205 (8.2%)
Fundus autofluorescence	253 (2.8%)/138 (5.5%)
Fluorescein angiography	70 (0.8%)/52 (2.1%)
Others	270 (3.0%)/162 (6.5%)

Among the patients who underwent baseline screening, 27.8% underwent subsequent monitoring examinations at any time after baseline. The mean number of monitoring examinations per year in those receiving monitoring examinations was found to be 0.68 ± 0.45, indicating a relatively low frequency of monitoring. The mean/median intervals from one examination to the subsequent examination were shortened from the baseline examination to the subsequent follow-up examinations. Similar to the baseline examinations, funduscopy/fundus photography was the most commonly employed modality for subsequent monitoring (98.6% utilization). OCT was used in 29.6% for the subsequent monitoring examinations, whereas other modalities were rarely used for baseline or monitoring examinations.

3.3. Trends of Retinopathy Screening among Tamoxifen Users over the Study Period

Table 4 presents the yearly trends in the proportion of tamoxifen users receiving retinopathy screening, including baseline examination and subsequent monitoring. From 2015 to 2020, the number of patients who underwent baseline examinations within 1 year gradually increased from 290 (4.6% among the annual users) in 2015 to 573 (7.7%) in 2020. Regarding subsequent monitoring, the percentage of patients examined within 6 months among those with baseline examinations ranged from 11.4% (in 2015) to 13.4% (in 2016) over the study period, while some fluctuations without a definite trend over time were noted. The percentage of patients monitored within 1 year of baseline screening among those with baseline examinations also showed a similar trend (Figure S2), with fluctuations ranging between 16.1% (in 2020) and 19.0% (in 2016).

Table 4. Yearly trends in the proportion of tamoxifen users undergoing retinopathy screening (baseline examination and subsequent monitoring).

Year	Baseline Examination within 1 Year	Monitoring	
		Examined within 6 Months from Baseline Exam (% among Those with Baseline)	Examined within 1 Year from Baseline Exam (% among Those with Baseline)
2015	290 (4.6%)	210 (11.4%)	286 (16.3%)
2016	411 (5.7%)	252 (13.4%)	358 (19.0%)
2017	453 (6.0%)	225 (12.9%)	302 (17.4%)
2018	524 (6.9%)	196 (13.2%)	268 (18.0%)
2019	585 (7.4%)	150 (11.7%)	221 (17.3%)
2020	573 (7.7%)	102 (12.5%)	131 (16.1%)

4. Discussion

This study aimed to investigate the trends and patterns of retinopathy screening among tamoxifen users in South Korea. Our analyses showed the population of tamoxifen users, performance and timing of baseline and subsequent monitoring examinations, and trends in retinopathy screening over the study period. Our data indicate that the frequency of monitoring was relatively low, with funduscopy/fundus photography being the preferred modality, followed by OCT. These findings suggest that screening practices for tamoxifen retinopathy should be enhanced to ensure regular and appropriate screening.

Regarding pathogenesis, tamoxifen retinopathy shares common features with Macular Telangiectasia type 2 (MacTel) [9,10], including telangiectasia of macular blood vessels and crystalline deposits in the macula, as highlighted by various studies [11,12]. These similarities suggest potential overlapping mechanisms in the development of tamoxifen retinopathy and MacTel type 2, warranting further investigation into their shared pathophysiology. For example, both conditions may involve vascular endothelial growth factor (VEGF) pathways and Muller cell defects in their pathogenesis, as suggested by recent research [9,10,13]. In addition, emerging evidence suggests a potential link between inflammation and tamoxifen-induced retinal changes [14], although further validation is needed to confirm this association. Moreover, there is a notable paucity of studies investigating biomarkers for tamoxifen retinopathy, highlighting the importance of research efforts aimed at identifying such markers for earlier detection and improved management strategies.

Analysis of annual trends in the number of tamoxifen users and initiators revealed a gradual increase over the study period. The total number of tamoxifen users was expected to reach 81,720 by 2021, representing 0.158% of the Korean population. Similarly, the number of patients initiating tamoxifen therapy has increased, reaching 18,012 by 2021. These findings suggest a growing population at a risk of tamoxifen-induced retinal toxicity in South Korea. As the number of tamoxifen users and initiators increases, it becomes crucial to establish effective retinopathy screening programs to ensure the early detection of potential retinal toxicity.

The study population consisted of 43,848 tamoxifen users, excluding those with prior ophthalmic diseases or conditions requiring retinopathy screening (i.e., diabetes mellitus), to include those requiring toxicity screening. Most users were female, consistent with the prevalent use of tamoxifen for breast cancer treatment. The mean age of the users was 45.0 years, with the highest proportion being 40–49 years old. The mean duration of tamoxifen use in our population was 36.0 months, indicating a significant period of medication exposure that is deemed sufficient to cause tamoxifen retinopathy according to the literature [2,15–17]. These data underscore the clinical significance of retinopathy screening for tamoxifen users, particularly in light of the escalating prevalence of breast cancer worldwide.

Our study identified several findings regarding the performance and timing of the baseline and subsequent monitoring examinations. Only a small proportion (6.5%) of tamoxifen users received baseline screening within 1 year of initiating therapy, indicating delayed or no referral to ophthalmologists for retinopathy screening. Remarkably, the overall proportion of patients undergoing any ophthalmic examination after tamoxifen use was only 20.4%, highlighting the need for increased awareness of tamoxifen-induced retinal toxicity and screening among prescribing physicians. By disseminating knowledge about the potential ocular side effects and the need for baseline and regular screening, ophthalmologists can raise awareness among prescribing physicians and promote appropriate referrals for screening examinations.

Funduscopy/fundus photography is the most commonly used modality for baseline screening and subsequent monitoring, indicating its widespread availability and ability to detect crystalline retinopathy with sensitivity [1,18]. However, the limited utilization of OCT shown in our data (21.9% at baseline and 29.6% for subsequent monitoring) may result in the failure to detect the subtle retinal changes associated with tamoxifen use [11,15]. For instance, tamoxifen retinopathy can present with pseudocystic foveal cavitation or photoreceptor disruption in OCT [2,19,20], in addition to typical refractile crystalline depositions in fundus photographs (crystalline retinopathy). Recent studies have shown a significant role of OCT in the sensitive detection of earlier changes, such as intraretinal pseudocysts and alterations of the photoreceptor layer [2,15,19,20]. Thus, our data suggest the need for the enhanced use of OCT for tamoxifen retinopathy screening. In light of this, the establishment of expert recommendations or guidelines emphasizing the utilization of OCT for tamoxifen retinopathy screening may be useful. In contrast, other modalities such as automated VF, FAF, and FA were rarely used, possibly reflecting their minor roles in retinopathy screening compared with funduscopy or OCT for tamoxifen users [1].

The frequency of subsequent monitoring examinations was relatively low, with a mean of 0.68 monitoring examinations per year. Furthermore, the percentage of patients receiving subsequent monitoring examinations within 1 year (annual examination) after the baseline examination was less than 20%. This finding implies that the frequency of monitoring should be increased and standardized. Ophthalmologists should contribute to ensuring the timely detection of retinopathy through several measures, including regular and timely monitoring and patient education/motivation for follow-up visits. Moreover, the analysis of the yearly trend in retinopathy screening among tamoxifen users further highlights the role of ophthalmologists in improving screening practices for tamoxifen retinopathy. For instance, although the proportion of patients undergoing baseline examinations within 1 year of tamoxifen use gradually increased, the percentage of patients examined within 6 months or 1 year after baseline screening fluctuated without a clear trend over time. This indicates an improvement in the timely initiation of retinopathy screening, which is mainly determined by prescribing physicians' referral to ophthalmologists, but no improvement in regular monitoring over time. Therefore, ophthalmologists should educate tamoxifen users about the importance of retinopathy screening, potential symptoms of retinal toxicity, and the significance of regular follow-up visits and motivate them to receive regular monitoring.

Additionally, ophthalmologists can contribute to the development and dissemination of evidence-based guidelines for screening for tamoxifen retinopathy. Specific guidelines may ensure consistent and standardized screening practices by ophthalmologists. For hydroxychloroquine, another well-known drug causing toxic retinopathy, recommendations for screening established by multiple organizations play significant roles in standardized screening practices and sensitive detection of the retinal toxicity [21,22]. In our previous study on hydroxychloroquine, there were significant improvements in timely baseline and annual monitoring over the same study period [8]. We believe that the difference in the presence of established guidelines between tamoxifen and hydroxychloroquine retinopathy might have led to the difference in the trend of screening practices over time between the two.

More specifically, for consistency and frequency of tamoxifen retinopathy screening, it is essential to establish a standardized protocol. This protocol should entail regular ophthalmologic evaluations for patients undergoing tamoxifen therapy, with initial screening at treatment initiation and subsequent follow-up examinations scheduled at regular intervals thereafter. Although the timing and frequency of screenings may vary based on factors such as treatment duration (or cumulative dosage) and individual risk factors, there is currently no consensus on the optimal schedule. However, a common recommendation is to conduct regular screenings including OCT, perhaps every 6 months, particularly for patients who have been on tamoxifen at a dosage of 20 mg/day for at least 2 years [1]. More frequent assessments may be warranted for individuals with higher risk profiles, preexisting ocular conditions, or symptomatic presentations. Effective collaboration between oncologists and ophthalmologists is imperative to ensure comprehensive and timely monitoring in patients undergoing tamoxifen therapy.

At present, there is no established consensus on the optimal treatment for tamoxifen-induced retinal toxicity. Discontinuing tamoxifen therapy should be considered as a preventative measure against further retinal damage. However, one promising approach involves the use of intravitreal steroids or anti-VEGF agents, similar to treatments employed for MacTel type 2 [1,23]. These medications have shown potential in alleviating pathological changes such as the cystic changes and macular edema commonly observed in tamoxifen retinopathy [1,24]. Additionally, it is important to address comorbidities such as hyperlipidemia and elevated body mass index as these have been linked to a higher risk of retinal changes with tamoxifen use [2]. Therefore, lowering lipid levels, promoting a low-fat diet and lifestyle modifications, might be beneficial in reducing the risk of retinal toxicity. Overall, further research is needed to fully understand the efficacy and safety of potential treatment modalities for tamoxifen-induced retinal toxicity and to develop novel therapies.

Although our study provides valuable insights into the trends and patterns of retinopathy screening among tamoxifen users, several limitations should be acknowledged when interpreting the results. First, it was conducted in South Korea, which may limit the generalizability of the findings to other populations with potentially different healthcare systems, cultural practices, and tamoxifen utilization patterns. Therefore, caution should be exercised when extrapolating these results to other populations. Second, our study relied on retrospective data obtained from the health claims database, which may include inherent limitations, such as missing or incorrect information, particularly in the diagnosis codes. Additionally, the study lacked information on the specific indications for ophthalmic examinations, which could have impacted the frequency and modality choices [25]. Finally, the study did not explore the reasons behind the observed trends in retinopathy screening or the potential barriers to screening practices. Understanding the factors influencing screening practices and identifying potential barriers to timely and adequate monitoring are crucial for developing targeted interventions and improving screening rates among tamoxifen users.

Another significant limitation of our study is the absence of an analysis of tamoxifen retinopathy cases. The lack of a specific diagnostic code for toxic maculopathy in the eighth revision of the Korean Standard Classification of Diseases hampered our ability to accurately identify all instances of tamoxifen retinopathy, potentially introducing bias. Moreover, tamoxifen retinopathy can manifest with diverse features like macular edema, which further complicates the interpretation of diagnostic codes. Although including the code for macular edema might enhance the detection of tamoxifen retinopathy cases, it also raises the risk of bias due to the other diverse causes of macular edema. Therefore, we intended to focus our analyses on investigating practice patterns for retinal toxicity and drug usage among tamoxifen users in this study rather than determining the precise incidence or prevalence of tamoxifen retinopathy.

5. Conclusions

Our study provides insights into the population of tamoxifen users, the performance of baseline and subsequent monitoring examinations, and trends in retinopathy screening over time. These findings highlight the need for continued efforts to optimize screening protocols, increase awareness among prescribing physicians and tamoxifen users, and improve the consistency and frequency of retinopathy screening in this at-risk population.

Supplementary Materials: The following supporting information can be downloaded at: https://www.mdpi.com/article/10.3390/jcm13082167/s1, Figure S1: Timing of baseline screening for tamoxifen retinopathy. The figure illustrates the timing of baseline screening for tamoxifen retinopathy, presented as the interval from the start date of tamoxifen treatment; Figure S2: Proportion of patients receiving baseline screening within 1 year of tamoxifen use and that of those with subsequent monitoring (within 1 year from the baseline examination) among those with baseline screening in each year between 2015 and 2020.

Author Contributions: Conceptualization, S.J.A.; methodology, S.J.A.; validation, S.J.A., J.K. and H.Y.K.; formal analysis, S.J.A., J.K. and H.Y.K.; investigation, S.J.A., J.K. and H.Y.K.; resources, S.J.A., J.K. and H.Y.K.; data curation, S.J.A., J.K. and H.Y.K.; writing—original draft preparation, S.J.A., J.K. and H.Y.K.; writing—review and editing, S.J.A.; visualization, S.J.A., J.K. and H.Y.K.; supervision, S.J.A.; project administration, S.J.A.; funding acquisition, S.J.A. All authors have read and agreed to the published version of the manuscript.

Funding: This work was supported by National Research Foundation of Korea grants (NRF-2021R1G1A1013360), funded by the Korean Government MSIT. Neither the sponsor nor the funding organization had any role in the design or conduct of this research.

Institutional Review Board Statement: This study was approved by the Institutional Review Board (IRB) of Hanyang University Hospital (IRB file number: 2023-01-003) on 10 January 2023.

Informed Consent Statement: The need/requirement for informed consent was waived by the IRB of Hanyang University Hospital because the retrospective study data were analyzed anonymously.

Data Availability Statement: Data are unavailable due to privacy and ethical restrictions.

Conflicts of Interest: The authors declare no conflicts of interest.

References

1. Bazvand, F.; Mahdizad, Z.; Mohammadi, N.; Shahi, F.; Mirghorbani, M.; Riazi-Esfahani, H.; Modjtahedi, B.S. Tamoxifen retinopathy. *Surv. Ophthalmol.* **2023**, *68*, 628–640. [CrossRef] [PubMed]
2. Kim, H.A.; Lee, S.; Eah, K.S.; Yoon, Y.H. Prevalence and Risk Factors of Tamoxifen Retinopathy. *Ophthalmology* **2020**, *127*, 555–557. [CrossRef] [PubMed]
3. Jordan, V.C. Fourteenth Gaddum Memorial Lecture. A current view of tamoxifen for the treatment and prevention of breast cancer. *Br. J. Pharmacol.* **1993**, *110*, 507–517. [CrossRef]
4. Vogel, V.G.; Costantino, J.P.; Wickerham, D.L.; Cronin, W.M.; Cecchini, R.S.; Atkins, J.N.; Bevers, T.B.; Fehrenbacher, L.; Pajon, E.R., Jr.; Wade, J.L., 3rd; et al. Effects of tamoxifen vs raloxifene on the risk of developing invasive breast cancer and other disease outcomes: The NSABP Study of Tamoxifen and Raloxifene (STAR) P-2 trial. *JAMA* **2006**, *295*, 2727–2741. [CrossRef] [PubMed]
5. Kaiser-Kupfer, M.I.; Kupfer, C.; Rodrigues, M.M. Tamoxifen retinopathy. A clinicopathologic report. *Ophthalmology* **1981**, *88*, 89–93. [CrossRef] [PubMed]
6. Kaiser-Kupfer, M.I.; Lippman, M.E. Tamoxifen retinopathy. *Cancer Treat. Rep.* **1978**, *62*, 315–320. [CrossRef] [PubMed]
7. Mauget-Faysse, M.; Gambrelle, J.; Quaranta-El Maftouhi, M. Optical coherence tomography in tamoxifen retinopathy. *Breast Cancer Res. Treat.* **2006**, *99*, 117–118. [CrossRef] [PubMed]
8. Kim, J.; Kim, K.E.; Kim, J.H.; Ahn, S.J. Practice Patterns of Screening for Hydroxychloroquine Retinopathy in South Korea. *JAMA Netw. Open* **2023**, *6*, e2314816. [CrossRef]
9. Moir, J.; Amin, S.V.; Khanna, S.; Komati, R.; Shaw, L.T.; Dao, D.; Hariprasad, S.M.; Skondra, D. Use of OCT Angiography to Diagnose and Manage Atypical Presentations of Macular Telangiectasia Type 2. *Int. J. Mol. Sci.* **2022**, *23*, 7849. [CrossRef]
10. Park, Y.J.; Lee, S.; Yoon, Y.H. One-year follow-up of optical coherence tomography angiography microvascular findings: Macular telangiectasia type 2 versus tamoxifen retinopathy. *Graefes Arch. Clin. Exp. Ophthalmol.* **2022**, *260*, 3479–3488. [CrossRef]
11. Lee, S.; Kim, H.A.; Yoon, Y.H. OCT Angiography Findings of Tamoxifen Retinopathy: Similarity with Macular Telangiectasia Type 2. *Ophthalmol. Retin.* **2019**, *3*, 681–689. [CrossRef]
12. Kovach, J.L.; Isildak, H.; Sarraf, D. Crystalline retinopathy: Unifying pathogenic pathways of disease. *Surv. Ophthalmol.* **2019**, *64*, 1–29. [CrossRef] [PubMed]
13. Charbel Issa, P.; Gillies, M.C.; Chew, E.Y.; Bird, A.C.; Heeren, T.F.; Peto, T.; Holz, F.G.; Scholl, H.P. Macular telangiectasia type 2. *Prog. Retin. Eye Res.* **2013**, *34*, 49–77. [CrossRef] [PubMed]

14. Wang, X.; Zhao, L.; Zhang, Y.; Ma, W.; Gonzalez, S.R.; Fan, J.; Kretschmer, F.; Badea, T.C.; Qian, H.H.; Wong, W.T. Tamoxifen Provides Structural and Functional Rescue in Murine Models of Photoreceptor Degeneration. *J. Neurosci.* **2017**, *37*, 3294–3310. [CrossRef] [PubMed]
15. Bolukbasi, S.; Kandemir Gursel, O.; Cakir, A.; Erden, B.; Karatas, G. Retinal structural changes in patients receiving tamoxifen therapy by spectral-domain optical coherence tomography. *Cutan. Ocul. Toxicol.* **2020**, *39*, 115–121. [CrossRef]
16. Crisostomo, S.; Vieira, L.; Cardigos, J.; Fernandes, D.H.; Luis, M.E.; Nunes, S.; Morujao, I.; Anjos, R.; Flores, R. TAMOXIFEN-INDUCED CHORIORETINAL CHANGES: An Optical Coherence Tomography and Optical Coherence Tomography Angiography Study. *Retina* **2020**, *40*, 1185–1190. [CrossRef]
17. Bicer, T.; Imamoglu, G.I.; Caliskan, S.; Bicer, B.K.; Gurdal, C. The Effects of Adjuvant Tamoxifen Use on Macula Pigment Epithelium Optical Density, Visual Acuity and Retinal Thickness in Patients with Breast Cancer. *Curr. Eye Res.* **2020**, *45*, 623–628. [CrossRef] [PubMed]
18. Gorin, M.B.; Day, R.; Costantino, J.P.; Fisher, B.; Redmond, C.K.; Wickerham, L.; Gomolin, J.E.; Margolese, R.G.; Mathen, M.K.; Bowman, D.M.; et al. Long-term tamoxifen citrate use and potential ocular toxicity. *Am. J. Ophthalmol.* **1998**, *125*, 493–501. [CrossRef] [PubMed]
19. Doshi, R.R.; Fortun, J.A.; Kim, B.T.; Dubovy, S.R.; Rosenfeld, P.J. Pseudocystic foveal cavitation in tamoxifen retinopathy. *Am. J. Ophthalmol.* **2014**, *157*, 1291–1298.e3. [CrossRef]
20. Gualino, V.; Cohen, S.Y.; Delyfer, M.N.; Sahel, J.A.; Gaudric, A. Optical coherence tomography findings in tamoxifen retinopathy. *Am. J. Ophthalmol.* **2005**, *140*, 757–758. [CrossRef]
21. Marmor, M.F.; Kellner, U.; Lai, T.Y.; Melles, R.B.; Mieler, W.F. Recommendations on Screening for Chloroquine and Hydroxychloroquine Retinopathy (2016 Revision). *Ophthalmology* **2016**, *123*, 1386–1394. [CrossRef] [PubMed]
22. Yusuf, I.H.; Foot, B.; Lotery, A.J. The Royal College of Ophthalmologists recommendations on monitoring for hydroxychloroquine and chloroquine users in the United Kingdom (2020 revision): Executive summary. *Eye* **2021**, *35*, 1532–1537. [CrossRef] [PubMed]
23. Jeng, K.W.; Wheatley, H.M. Intravitreal triamcinolone acetonide treatment of tamoxifen maculopathy with associated cystoid macular edema. *Retin. Cases Brief. Rep.* **2015**, *9*, 64–66. [CrossRef] [PubMed]
24. Li, C.; Xiao, J.; Zou, H.; Yang, B.; Luo, L. The response of anti-VEGF therapy and tamoxifen withdrawal of tamoxifen-induced cystoid macular edema in the same patient. *BMC Ophthalmol.* **2021**, *21*, 201. [CrossRef]
25. Kim, J.; Kwon, H.Y.; Kim, J.H.; Ahn, S.J. Nationwide Usage of Pentosan Polysulfate and Practice Patterns of Pentosan Polysulfate Maculopathy Screening in South Korea. *Ophthalmol. Retin.* **2024**, *8*, 246–253. [CrossRef]

Journal of
Clinical Medicine

MDPI

Article

Autosomal Dominant Retinitis Pigmentosa Secondary to TOPORS Mutations: A Report of a Novel Mutation and Clinical Findings

Alen T. Eid [1,*], Kevin Toni Eid [2], James Vernon Odom [1], David Hinkle [3] and Monique Leys [1,*]

1 Department of Ophthalmology and Visual Sciences, West Virginia University School of Medicine, Morgantown, WV 26506, USA; jodom@hsc.wvu.edu
2 Department of Ophthalmology and Visual Sciences, John A. Moran Eye Center, University of Utah, Salt Lake City, UT 84112, USA; keid@oakland.edu
3 Tulane University School of Medicine, New Orleans, LA 70112, USA; davidhinklemd@gmail.com
* Correspondence: ateid@umich.edu (A.T.E.); leysm@wvumedicine.org (M.L.)

Abstract: Purpose: Mutations in Topoisomerase I–binding RS protein (TOPORS) have been previously documented and have been described to result in pathological autosomal dominant retinitis pigmentosa (adRP). In our study, we describe the various genotypes and clinical/phenotypic manifestations of TOPORS-related mutations of our unique patient population in Rural Appalachia. **Methods:** The medical records of 416 patients with inherited retinal disease at the West Virginia University Eye Institute who had undergone genetic testing between the years of 2015–2022 were reviewed. Patients found to have pathologic RP and mutations related to TOPORS were then analyzed. **Results:** In total, 7 patients (ages 12–70) were identified amongst three unique families. All patients were female in our study. The average follow-up period was 7.7 years. A mother (70 yr) and daughter (51 yr) had a novel heterozygous nonsense point mutation in TOPORS c.2431C > T, p.Gln811X (Exon 3) that led to premature termination of the desired protein resulting in early onset vision loss, cataract formation, and visual field restriction. The mother developed a full-thickness macular hole which was successfully repaired. Five other patients were found to have previously described TOPORS mutations. Visual field loss was progressive with age in both cohorts. **Conclusions:** Seven patients at our institution were identified to have mutations in TOPORS resulting in autosomal dominant retinitis pigmentosa. Two patients were found to have novel truncating mutations in the TOPORS gene resulting in profound night blindness and visual field loss, recurrent macular edema, and in one individual, epiretinal membrane formation leading to a macular hole which was able to be successfully repaired.

Keywords: TOPORS; retinitis pigmentosa; OCT; retina; ADRP; Appalachia; inherited retinal disease; retinal degeneration; RP; genetics; mutation; macular hole

1. Introduction

Retinitis pigmentosa (RP) is a group of inherited retinal dystrophies characterized by the progressive degeneration of photoreceptors and retinal pigment epithelium (RPE), leading to night blindness, visual field constriction, and eventual loss of central vision. RP affects approximately 1 in 4000 individuals worldwide and is genetically heterogeneous, with more than 80 genes implicated in its pathogenesis [1–3]. Autosomal dominant RP (adRP) accounts for about 15–30% of all RP cases and is caused by mutations in at least 25 genes [1,3,4].

One of the genes associated with adRP is TOPORS, which encodes topoisomerase I-binding RS protein, a dual E3 ubiquitin and SUMO1 nuclear protein ligase that is involved in cell cycle regulation, protein synthesis, DNA repair, and chromatin modification in different cell types [3–6]. The gene itself is present on the short arm of chromosome 9 band 21, is roughly 12,000 base pairs in length, and encodes a ubiquitous multidomain SUMO1-Protein E3 ligase protein comprised of 3 exons. Mutations in TOPORS have been reported to cause adRP linked to chromosome 9p21.1 (locus RP31) in several families from different ethnic backgrounds. Pathologic mutations in the retina eventually lead to loss of the outer portions of the photoreceptors which is likely related to the disruption of cilia-dependent photoreceptor cell maintenance pathways [4,7]. The majority of these mutations are located in the terminal half of exon 3 and result in premature truncation or missense changes of the TOPORS protein.

The phenotypic features of TOPORS-related RP may include early onset of night blindness, severe progressive visual field constriction, cystoid maculopathy (CM), and reduced electroretinogram (ERG) stimulatory responses. Given the rare nature of TOPORS-related RP, genotype–phenotype correlations of TOPORS mutations and the exact molecular mechanisms behind retinal degeneration caused by TOPORS dysfunction are still not fully understood [3].

In this case, we report the prevalence and characterization of TOPORS mutations in a cohort of patients with inherited retinal disease from rural Appalachia. We identified seven patients from three separate families with mutations in TOPORS, including the identification of a novel nonsense mutation that causes premature truncation of the protein. Their clinical course and examination findings are described in detail below. Lastly, we describe an isolated case of full thickness macular hole that was successfully repaired and was able to restore limited vision in one of our patients with TOPORS-related RP. A preliminary review of the research gathered from this study was presented at the 2023 ARVO Annual Meeting in New Orleans, LA.

2. Methods

2.1. Patient Population

We performed a retrospective review of 416 patients who were diagnosed with inherited retinal disease at the WVU Eye Institute from January 2015 to June 2023. Most patients underwent comprehensive ophthalmic examination, including best-corrected visual acuity (BCVA), slit-lamp biomicroscopy, fundus photography, optical coherence tomography (OCT), visual field testing, and electrophysiology testing. The diagnosis of TOPORS related retinitis pigmentosa was based on clinical findings and confirmatory genetic testing. The study was approved by the Institutional Review Board of West Virginia University.

2.2. Genetic Analysis

Confirmatory genetic testing was completed at three different laboratories. Blueprint Genetics (MyRetinaTracker; Helsinki, Finland) with support from Foundation Fighting Blindness (Columbia, MD, USA), Invitae (ID Your IRD panel; San Francisco, CA, USA) with support from Spark Therapeutics (Philadelphia, PA, USA), and the Laboratory for Molecular Diagnosis of Inherited Eye Diseases (LMDIED Human Genetics Center—Houston, TX, USA) with support from The National Ophthalmic Disease Genotyping and Phenotyping Network eyeGENE NEI (Bethesda, MD, USA).

Samples processed by Blueprint Genetics were sequenced via high-quality custom capture technology and next-generation sequencing (NGS) for the IRB study protocol panel of 322 genes. Samples processed by Invitae were sequenced through similar technologies as part of a 248 to 330 gene panel. Confirmatory sequence analysis for samples processed by LMDIED were tested against a limited 9 gene panel for common mutations responsible for adRP after preliminary screening through eyeGENE at NEI. The members of Family 1 (F1) underwent testing with Blueprint Genetics. The members of Family 2 (F2) underwent testing with Invitae. Lastly, the members of Family 3 underwent testing with LMDIED. Within F3, Patient 7 (F7) underwent dual testing with LMDIED and Invitae.

3. Results

3.1. Identification of TOPORS Mutations

Among the 416 patients with inherited retinal disease at our institution, we identified a total of 7 patients from three separate families who had mutations in TOPORS (Figure 1). All identified patients were female and initially presented to our clinic with ages ranging from 12 to 70 years of age. A total of 7 out of 7 patients underwent confirmatory genetic testing. The average follow-up time in our patient population was (7.7 years). All mutations were heterozygous and segregated with the disease phenotype in each family.

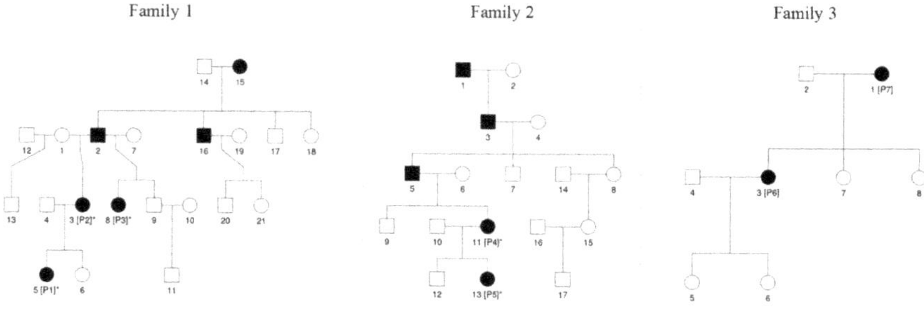

Figure 1. Shown above is the pedigree for the three study populations. All families demonstrate autosomal dominant inheritance patterns found in TOPORS related retinitis pigmentosa. The "*" represents probands with known mutational variants.

Of the study population, two families (F1 and F2) were found to have a previously reported frameshift mutation at c.2556_2557del (p.Glu852fs) that introduces a premature stop codon at position 871. One family (F3) had a novel nonsense mutation c.2431C>T (p.Gln811X) that replaces a glutamine codon into a stop codon at position 811.

3.2. Clinical Features of Patients with TOPORS Mutations

The exam findings and clinical characteristics of the 7 patients with TOPORS mutations are summarized in Table 1. Of note, missing data points are the result of incomplete documentation or loss to follow-up during retrospective chart review using the institutions electronic medical record. For symptomatic individuals, the average age of onset for vision loss was in their early 20's. The most common complaint was night blindness, followed by progressive loss of peripheral vision and central vision in symptomatic individuals. The BCVA at the time of last follow up ranged from 20/20 to 20/60.

Fundus examination revealed typical RP features, such as bone spicule pigmentation, attenuated retinal vessels, optic disc pallor, and macular changes (Figure 2). There was significant thinning of the outer nuclear layer and disruption of the ellipsoid zone in all patients who underwent spectral domain OCT (SD-OCT) testing. CM was only present in two patients (P6 and P7). Patient P7 suffered from chronic bilateral vitreomacular traction (VMT) that eventually led to the development of a full thickness macular hole leading to rapid vision loss throughout the follow-up period. When available, all patients undergoing fundus autofluorescence photography (FAF) demonstrated diffuse reduced peripheral retina autofluorescence with a central fluorescent ring within the area of the macula correlating to remaining island of functional central photoreceptors at the fovea as seen in Figure 3. Visual field defects vary between individuals and the severity of peripheral vision loss correlated with age and the stage of the of RP. The visual field testing for P6 and P3 are shown below. In addition to abnormal FAF, ERG changes were documented in a subset of our patients who were able to undergo testing. Figure 4 demonstrates diminished full field ERG testing in P4 in primary in a dark-adapted scotopic environment consistent with the chief complaint of night blindness.

Table 1. A relative overview of demographics from the study population. Unavailable or incomplete information is listed with "NA". ADHD = Attention-Defcit/Hyperactivity Disorder. GAD = Generalized Anxiety Disorder. IBS = Irritable Bowel Syndrome. GERD = Gastroesophageal Reflux Disease. PSC = Posterior Subcapsular Cataract. CME = Cystoid Macular Edema. PCIOL = Posterior Chamber Intraocular Lens. ERM = Epiretinal Membrane. FTMH = Full-Thickness Macular Hole. PTMH = Partial Thickness Macular Hole. GVF = Goldmann Visual Field.

ID	Family	Sex	Age at Last Follow Up	Age of Onset	Follow Up Time	Past Medical History	Past Ocular History	TOPORS Mutational Variant	BCVA OD	BCVA OS	Visual Field Testing
P1	F1	F	12	NA	2 Years	Autism, ADHD, Gait abnormality	None	c.2556_2557del	20/30 − 1	20/25 + 2	Mild Restriction OD. Smallest target seen is I3e.
P2	F1	F	35	20 s	2 Years	GAD, Smoker	Dry Eye	c.2556_2557del	20/25 1	20/40	NA
P3	F1	F	32	18	13 Years	IBS, GAD, Endometriosis	None	c.2556_2557del	20/25 − 1	20/25 − 1	About 80 central vision OU. Smallest target seen is V4e OD and I4e OS.
P4	F2	F	43	20 s	4 Years	GERD, Hypothyroidism	PSC OU	c.2556_2557del	20/25 − 1	20/25 − 1	Ring scotoma OU. Smallest target seen is I4e.
P5	F2	F	25	20 s	2 Months	GAD	Photophobia	c.2556_2557del	20/20	20/20	NA
P6	F3	F	51	20s	17 Years	Nephrolithiasis, Smoker, GAD	PSC OD, CME OU, PCIOL OD	c.2431C>T	20/60 − 1	20/60 + 2	GVF OU limited to central 10 degrees. Smallest target is I4e.
P7	F3	F	70	20 s	16 Years	Nephrolithiasis, Hypertension, Hyperlipidemia	PCIOL OU, Hx of PSC OU, CME OU, ERM OU, FTMH OD, PTMH OS	c.2431C>T	20/60	20/40	GVF of less than 10 degrees OU. Smallest target seen is V4e.

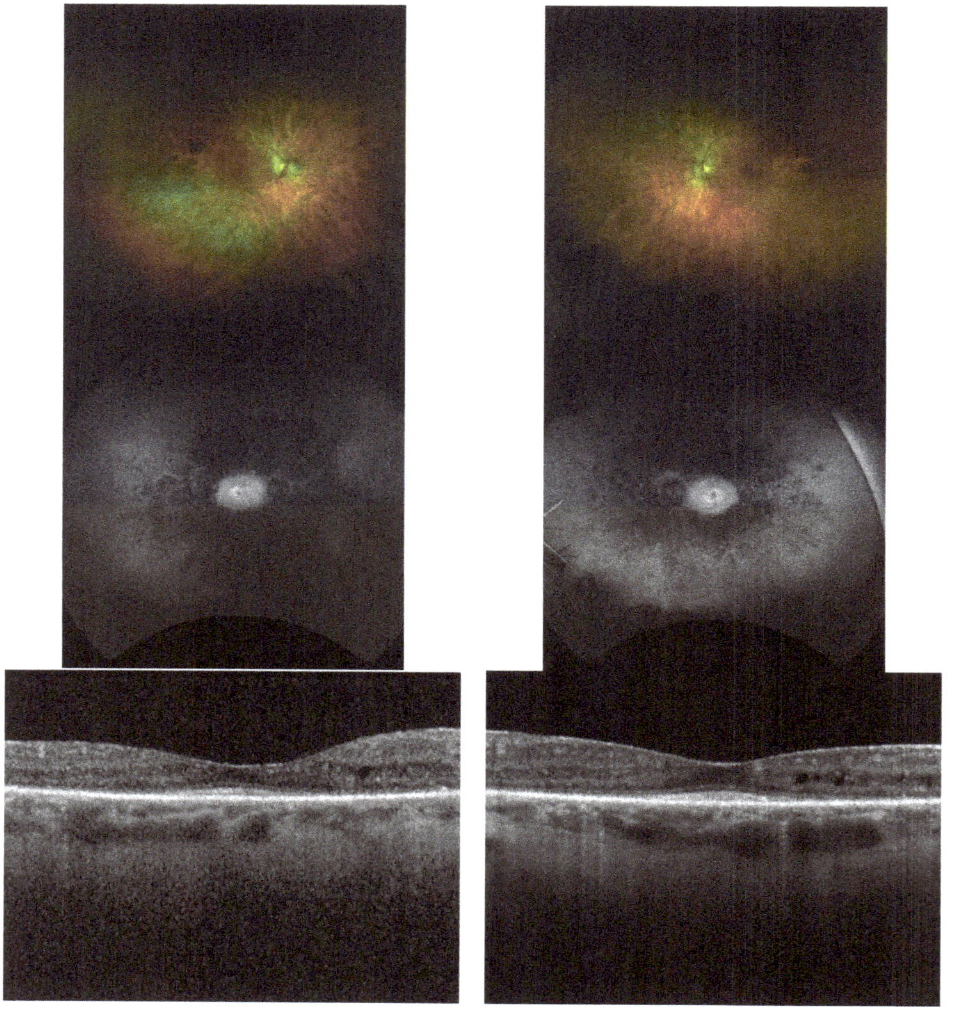

Figure 2. Ultra-Wide Field Fundus Images with FAF and OCT of the macula in P6 (Right Column—Right Eye, Left Column—Left Eye. The classic triad waxy optic nerve pallor, vascular attenuation, and bone spicules are all demonstrated in this image series. Notice the reduced peripheral fundus autofluorescence with a preserved central island in the macula. OCT findings of the macula demonstrate cystoid maculopathy with diffuse loss of the ellipsoid zone and outer retinal thinning.

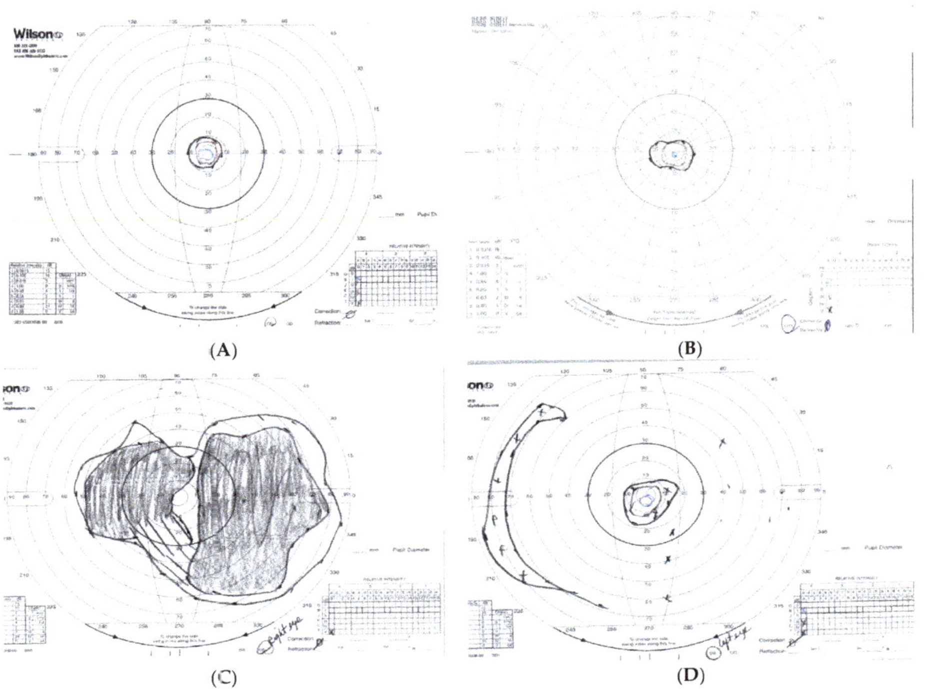

Figure 3. Goldmann Visual fields for P6 (above: (**A**)—Right Eye, (**B**)—Left Eye) and P3 (below: (**C**)—Right Eye, (**D**)—Left Eye). Notice the diffuse progressive loss in peripheral vision in both patients.

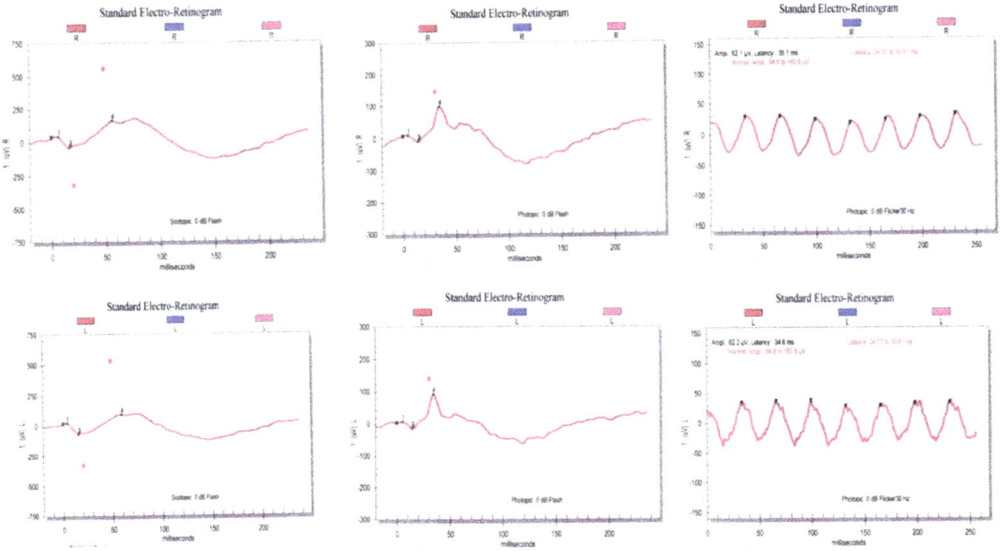

Figure 4. Full—field ERG demonstrating reduced a and b waves in a dark and light adapted setting ins subject P4. A wave amplitude is markedly attenuated which is consistent with the patients diminished photoreceptor function (Top—Right Eye, Bottom—Left Eye).

3.3. An Isolated Case of Full Thickness Macular Hole Leading to Rapid Vision Loss with Successful Repair

Within the subset of our patients with symptomatic RP secondary to TOPORS mutations, we report a 70-year-old female patient (P7) who developed a full thickness macular hole (FTMH) in her right eye measuring approximately 230 μm. The patient had a history of chronic vision loss in both eyes since the age of 30 years old. She also had a history of CM for years with concomitant VMT, which was refractory to topical carbonic anhydrase inhibitors and a series of intravitreal steroid injections. Genetic testing revealed that she carried the novel c.2431C>T (p.Gln811X) TOPORS mutation.

At the time of presentation for her full FTMH, her best corrected visual acuity (BCVA) was found to be 20/60 − 1 in the right eye and 20/50 − 1 in the left. She underwent 25-gauge pars plana vitrectomy (PPV) with epiretinal membrane (ERM) peel, internal limiting membrane (ILM) peel, and sulfur hexafluoride (SF6) gas tamponade with 7-day face down positioning in both eyes.

In the first OCT sequence (Figure 5), the patient presented with a full thickness macular hole measuring 230 μm in diameter in the right eye. Her BCVA was 20/60 − 1 and her Goldmann visual field (GVF) showed less than the central 10° in the affected eye. In the third sequence, one year after the surgery, the macular hole was closed and the foveal contour was restored in the right eye. Her BCVA improved to 20/40 and she reported subjective improvement in central metamorphopsia which was also demonstrated on interval Amsler gird testing. The macular hole was found to remain closed at the time of her 3-year follow up.

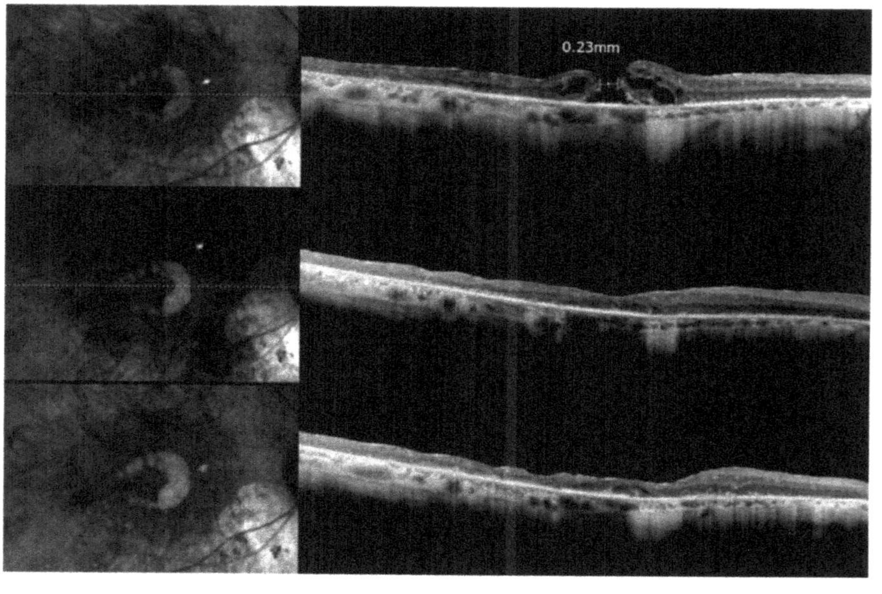

Figure 5. Spectral Domain OCT series of the right macula in P7. The first sequence (**top**) demonstrates the presence of a full thickness macular hole with adjacent cystoid macular edema and a faint epiretinal membrane. The second (**middle**) sequence was taken 1 month following the patient macular hole repair via pars plana vitrectomy with ERM and ILM peeling. In the third and final (**bottom**) sequence, we can appreciate persistent surgical closure of the full thickness macular hole 1 year following surgery. In all image series, there is diffuse outer retinal atrophy and photoreceptor loss consistent with late-stage retinitis pigmentosa.

4. Discussion

Mutations in TOPORS are a rare cause of autosomal dominant retinitis pigmentosa, with only a few families reported worldwide. In this study, we identified 7 patients from 3 families with TOPORS mutations in a cohort of 416 patients with inherited retinal disease from rural Appalachia treated at our institution. This represents the prevalence of TOPORs related RP to be 1.68% of adRP cases in our cohort similar to the estimated prevalence of 1% reported by Daiger, further emphasizing the rare nature of TOPORs related disease [1].

We identified a novel nonsense mutation c.2431C>T (p.Gln811X) in one family (F3), which is predicted to replace a glutamine codon with a stop codon, truncating the TOPORS protein by about 233 amino acids. Similar to previously described mutations, early truncation of the protein within exon 3 leads to deterioration of the Really Interesting New Gene (RING) finger motif function that is essential for ubiquitin ligase activity. Previous studies have shown that mutations in this domain impair the ubiquitination and degradation of p53, a tumor suppressor protein that regulates cell cycle and apoptosis [5]. It is possible that this mutation affects the stability and function of p53 in photoreceptors, leading to their degeneration. This mutation also agrees with the finding by Wang et al. that amino acid residues damaged at positions 807 to 867 which results in pathologic TOPORS phenotypes [8]. At the time of publication, only one other similar mutation reported by Invitae to NIH's ClinVar database has been documented at c.2431C>G (p.Gln811Glu). This single nucleotide mutation has been described at the same location which replaces a glutamine with glutamic acid residue at the 811 position, which as of now is listed as a mutation of uncertain significance [9].

The two other families (F1, F2) had a previously reported frameshift mutation c.2556_2557del (p.Glu852fs), which is one of the most common TOPORS mutations found in adRP patients [1,7,10]. This nonsense mutation also results in a premature stop codon at position 871, which may lead to early degradation of the mRNA or a truncated protein with an absent RING finger domain.

The clinical features of our patients with TOPORS mutations appear to be consistent with previous reports of TOPORS-related RP. In most cases, disease onset was early, with night blindness being the first symptom. Similar to other aggressive RP, progression was severe, with the loss of peripheral then central vision leading to legal blindness by the fifth or sixth decade of life. Fundus appearance was also consistent with that of typical RP, such as bone spicule pigmentation, vessel attenuation, optic disc pallor, and pigmentary macular changes. On SD-OCT, findings revealed thinning of the outer nuclear layer and irregularity of the ellipsoid zone indicating photoreceptor loss. The visual field defects varied between individuals and the severity of peripheral vision loss correlated with age and the stage of the RP.

CM was present in two patients (P6 and P7). This appears to be a common complication of RP that can affect visual acuity and quality of life in patients with already limited vison. Interestingly enough, CM was not seen in the other families. Diabetes and other renal dysfunctions which are known independent causes of CM formation were not comorbid conditions in our study group. This may suggest that the patients in novel mutation group (F3) may be more predisposed to CM formation. However, further evidence to support this claim may be confounded by VMT or other variables not accounted for in our analysis. CME typically can be treated with topical or systemic anti-inflammatory agents, carbonic anhydrase inhibitors, or other intravitreal injections [11]. However, treatment response is variable depending on the severity of disease and often affected by other underlying comorbidities.

In our study group, one patient developed a full thickness macular hole (FTMH), which can be a rare occurrence in RP patients. FTMH is primarily a byproduct of abnormal vitreomacular forces [12]. It is characterized by a defect in the foveal neurosensory retina that extends through all retinal layers and causes detrimental central vision loss. The pathogenesis of FTMH in RP patients is not well understood, but has been previously described to be related to chronic VMT, ERM formation, or retinal atrophy [13,14]. FTMH can be surgically repaired by PPV with ILM peeling and supplemental gas tamponade. Repair of macular holes in RP patient is rare and long-term outcomes are poorly understood [13,14]. As in the case of our patient (P7), we performed a successful repair of a FTMH surgery, which resulted in improved visual acuity and persistent primary surgical success given persistent closure of the macular hole over three years of follow up.

The exact function of TOPORS in the retina is still unknown. Prior research has demonstrated TOPORS importance in maintaining photoreceptor homeostasis and survival through its supportive ubiquitin and SUMO1 ligase activities [5,6,15]. Mutations in TOPORS cause an aggressive form of RP compared to other adRP genes, which may reflect its involvement in multiple cellular pathways and processes as previously described. Further studies are needed to define the exact pathologic mechanisms underlying TOPORS-related RP and to identify potential therapeutic targets.

At the time of publication, the c.2431C>T (p.Gln811X) mutational variant demonstrated in F3 was recently changed in classification from a variant of uncertain significance (VUS) to "Likely Pathogenic" by Invitae in the latest report received in December 2023. Family 3 was affected by this variant had demonstrated early onset and aggressive RP in our study. Not all variants present in a gene cause disease, and some may be benign polymorphisms [2,9,15–18]. Similar to prior studies, premature translational stop signals in TOPORS related RP at exon 3 have shown to be pathologic, which provides additional evidence for the pathogenicity of our novel mutation [8].

5. Conclusions

In conclusion, we report the prevalence and characterization of TOPORS related RP mutations in a cohort of patients with inherited retinal disease from rural Appalachia. In our study population, we identified a novel nonsense TOPORS mutation c.2431C>T (p.Gln811X) in one family and a previously described frameshift mutation c.2556_2557del(p.Glu852fs) in two other unrelated families with pathologic adRP. Both of these mutations would appear to truncate the TOPORS protein and impair its E3 ubiquitin ligase activity, which may affect the stability and function of supportive cell cycle regulatory proteins in photoreceptors. We were also able to confirm that TOPORS-related RP is an early onset and severe form of RP that leads to legal blindness by the fifth or sixth decade of life in our unique study population.

The fundus appearance, OCT findings, ERG responses, and visual field defects were consistent with typical RP. CM was present in two patients and FTMH was present in one patient. We also describe a case of successful FTMH surgery in one of our patients with the novel mutational variant (P6), which resulted in improved visual acuity and persistent anatomical closure of the macular hole after three years of follow up. Our findings expand on the existing fund of knowledge related to the genetic and phenotypic spectrum of TOPORS-related RP, providing insights into its pathogenesis and management. Further studies are needed to elucidate the molecular mechanisms underlying TOPORS-related RP and to identify a potential for therapeutic targets or the possibility of gene therapy in the relative future.

Author Contributions: Investigation, J.V.O., D.H. and M.L.; Writing—original draft, A.T.E.; Writing—review & editing, K.T.E. and M.L.; Supervision, J.V.O., D.H. and M.L.; Project administration, D.H. All authors have read and agreed to the published version of the manuscript.

Funding: This research received no external funding.

Institutional Review Board Statement: This research study was granted an exemption in accordance with Research on existing data, documents, records, pathological specimens, or diagnostic specimens [45 CFR 46.101(4)] by the Institutional Review Board.

Informed Consent Statement: Not applicable.

Data Availability Statement: Not applicable.

Acknowledgments: Our sincere thanks to Regina Starn, C.O.A, for her dedicated service in visual field testing and contributions to our clinic's success over the years.

Conflicts of Interest: The authors declare no conflict of interest.

References

1. Bowne, S.J.; Sullivan, L.S.; Gire, A.I.; Birch, D.G.; Hughbanks-Wheaton, D.; Heckenlively, J.R.; Daiger, S.P. Mutations in the *TOPORS* gene cause 1% of autosomal dominant retinitis pigmentosa. *Mol. Vis.* **2008**, *14*, 922–927. [PubMed]
2. Schob, C.; Orth, U.; Gal, A.; Kindler, S.; Chakarova, C.F.; Bhattacharya, S.S.; Rüther, K. Mutations in TOPORS: A Rare Cause of Autosomal Dominant Retinitis Pigmentosa in Continental Europe? *Ophthalmic Genet.* **2009**, *30*, 96–98. [CrossRef] [PubMed]
3. He, K.; Zhou, Y.; Li, N. Mutations of TOPORS identified in families with retinitis pigmentosa. *Ophthalmic Genet.* **2022**, *43*, 371–377. [CrossRef] [PubMed]
4. Chakarova, C.F.; Khanna, H.; Shah, A.Z.; Patil, S.B.; Sedmak, T.; Murga-Zamalloa, C.A.; Papaioannou, M.G.; Nagel-Wolfrum, K.; Lopez, I.; Munro, P.; et al. TOPORS, implicated in retinal degeneration, is a cilia-centrosomal protein. *Hum. Mol. Genet.* **2011**, *20*, 975. [CrossRef] [PubMed]
5. Saleem, A.; Dutta, J.; Malegaonkar, D.; Rasheed, F.; Rasheed, Z.; Rajendra, R.; Marshall, H.; Luo, M.; Li, H.; Rubin, E.H. The topoisomerase I- and p53-binding protein topors is differentially expressed in normal and malignant human tissues and may function as a tumor suppressor. *Oncogene* **2004**, *23*, 5293–5300. [CrossRef] [PubMed]
6. Rajendra, R.; Malegaonkar, D.; Pungaliya, P.; Marshall, H.; Rasheed, Z.; Brownell, J.; Liu, L.F.; Lutzker, S.; Saleem, A.; Rubin, E.H. Topors functions as an E3 ubiquitin ligase with specific E2 enzymes and ubiquitinates p53. *J. Biol. Chem.* **2004**, *279*, 36440–36444. [CrossRef] [PubMed]
7. Chakarova, C.F.; Papaioannou, M.G.; Khanna, H.; Lopez, I.; Waseem, N.; Shah, A.; Theis, T.; Friedman, J.; Maubaret, C.; Bujakowska, K.; et al. Mutations in TOPORS Cause Autosomal Dominant Retinitis Pigmentosa with Perivascular Retinal Pigment Epithelium Atrophy. *Am. J. Hum Genet.* **2007**, *81*, 1098–1103. [CrossRef] [PubMed]
8. Wang, J.; Wang, Y.; Jiang, Y.; Li, X.; Xiao, X.; Li, S.; Jia, X.; Sun, W.; Wang, P.; Zhang, Q. Autosomal Dominant Retinitis Pigmentosa–Associated TOPORS Protein Truncating Variants Are Exclusively Located in the Region of Amino Acid Residues 807 to 867. *Investig. Opthalmol. Vis. Sci.* **2022**, *63*, 19. [CrossRef] [PubMed]
9. VCV001510617.4—ClinVar—NCBI. Available online: https://www.ncbi.nlm.nih.gov/clinvar/variation/1510617/ (accessed on 9 May 2023).
10. Coussa, R.G.; Chakarova, C.; Ajlan, R.; Taha, M.; Kavalec, C.; Gomolin, J.; Khan, A.; Lopez, I.; Ren, H.; Waseem, N.; et al. Genotype and Phenotype Studies in Autosomal Dominant Retinitis Pigmentosa (adRP) of the French Canadian Founder Population. *Investig. Ophthalmol. Vis. Sci.* **2015**, *56*, 8297–8305. [CrossRef] [PubMed]
11. Genead, M.A.; Fishman, G.A. Efficacy of sustained topical dorzolamide therapy for cystic macular lesions in patients with retinitis pigmentosa and usher syndrome. *Arch. Ophthalmol. Ill 1960* **2010**, *128*, 1146–1150. [CrossRef]
12. Duker, J.S.; Kaiser, P.K.; Binder, S.; de Smet, M.D.; Gaudric, A.; Reichel, E.; Sadda, S.R.; Sebag, J.; Spaide, R.F.; Stalmans, P. The International Vitreomacular Traction Study Group classification of vitreomacular adhesion, traction, and macular hole. *Ophthalmology* **2013**, *120*, 2611–2619. [CrossRef]
13. Giusti, C.; Forte, R.; Vingolo, E.M. Clinical pathogenesis of macular holes in patients affected by retinitis pigmentosa. *Eur. Rev. Med. Pharmacol. Sci.* **2002**, *6*, 45–48. [PubMed]
14. Lee, C.Y.; Yang, C.M.; Yang, C.H.; Hu, F.R.; Chen, T.C. Flap technique-assisted surgeries for advanced retinitis pigmentosa complicated with macular hole: A case report and literature review. *BMC Ophthalmol.* **2021**, *21*, 322. [CrossRef] [PubMed]
15. All Variants in the TOPORS Gene—Global Variome Shared LOVD. Available online: https://databases.lovd.nl/shared/variants/TOPORS?search_position_c_start=2556&search_position_c_start_intron=0&search_position_c_end=2557&search_position_c_end_intron=0&search_vot_clean_dna_change==%22c.2556_2557del%22&search_transcriptid=00021645 (accessed on 15 May 2023).
16. Unique Variants in the TOPORS Gene—Global Variome Shared LOVD. Available online: https://databases.lovd.nl/shared/variants/TOPORS/unique (accessed on 9 May 2023).
17. Sullivan, L.S.; Bowne, S.J.; Reeves, M.J.; Blain, D.; Goetz, K.; NDifor, V.; Vitez, S.; Wang, X.; Tumminia, S.J.; Daiger, S.P. Prevalence of mutations in eyeGENE probands with a diagnosis of autosomal dominant retinitis pigmentosa. *Investig. Ophthalmol. Vis. Sci.* **2013**, *54*, 6255–6261. [CrossRef] [PubMed]
18. TOPORS | gnomAD v2.1.1 | gnomAD. Available online: https://gnomad.broadinstitute.org/gene/ENSG00000197579?dataset=gnomad_r2_1 (accessed on 4 June 2023).

Journal of
Clinical Medicine

MDPI

Article

Fixed Quarterly Dosing of Aflibercept after Loading Doses in Neovascular Age-Related Macular Degeneration in Chinese Eyes

Daniel H. T. Wong [1,2,3] and Kenneth K. W. Li [1,2,3,*]

1 Department of Ophthalmology, United Christian Hospital, Hospital Authority, Hong Kong, China
2 Department of Ophthalmology, Tseung Kwan O Hospital, Hospital Authority, Hong Kong, China
3 Department of Ophthalmology, School of Clinical Medicine, LKS Faculty of Medicine, The University of Hong Kong, Hong Kong, China
* Correspondence: kennethli@rcsed.ac.uk; Tel.: +852-3949-3411

Abstract: We aimed to investigate the success rate of planned fixed quarterly aflibercept injections after three loading doses (QDA3L) to achieve stability without recurrence in neovascular age-related macular degeneration (nAMD) at a tertiary eye centre. A retrospective study was conducted over five years (2017–2021) by including all consecutive cases of nAMD treated with three initial aflibercept injections four weeks apart, followed by planned injection appointments every 12 to 16 weeks starting from week 20. The primary endpoint was to determine the proportion of patients who maintained disease inactivity at week 52 and week 104. A total of 40 eyes of 40 patients were included. The overall mean age was 80.8, with a male preponderance. The overall success rate in our study population was 52.9% and 53.6% at week 52 and week 104, respectively. The fovea remained dry at 85.3% at week 52 and 82.1% at week 104, and 85.3% and 85.7% of subjects lost fewer than 15 ETDRS letters at week 52 and week 104, respectively. While this study does not suggest the superiority of this regimen, the success and failure rates obtained in our study can be used in the counselling process for this particular fixed treatment regimen for nAMD.

Keywords: anti-VEGF; macular degeneration; aflibercept; treat and extend; quarterly injections

1. Introduction

1.1. Anti-Vascular Endothelial Growth Factors and the Global Treatment Burden

Age-related macular degeneration (AMD) accounts for 8.7% of all causes of blindness worldwide and is the most common cause of blindness in developed nations [1]. Its prevalence is likely to increase as a consequence of exponential population ageing [1]. The estimated population suffering from AMD worldwide was 196 million in 2020, projected to increase to 288 million by 2040 [1]. Wet, or neovascular, AMD affects 10–15% of AMD patients and is characterised by macular neovascularisation (MNV), where new immature blood vessels grow towards the outer retina, typically from the underlying choroid, resulting in leakage, fluid accumulation, and haemorrhage [2]. Vascular endothelial growth factors (VEGF), as proangiogenic messengers, play a significant role in neovascularisation [2]. Anti-vascular endothelial growth factors (Anti-VEGF) are important medications regarded as the gold standard used to treat neovascular age-related macular degeneration (nAMD) [3]. One of the main goals of anti-VEGF treatment regimens is to minimise the fluctuations of central subfield thickness of the macula to improve functional outcomes [3–5]. Different treatment regimens exist, including the pro re nata (PRN) and the treat and extend (T&E) approaches. The T&E regimen was thought by experts to be more proactive and personalised and is associated with decreased treatment and monitoring burden, better utilisation of clinical resources, and minimisation of the risk of visual loss [3].

Treating macular disease with anti-VEGF has been an enormous burden to ophthalmic services globally. Hong Kong is not an exception. Treatment burden involves frequent clinic visits, travel, emotional burden, caregiver support, appointment booking, visual acuity checks, fundus imaging, financial burden for the patients, and workload for the staff involved in administering the injections [6]. In Hong Kong, anti-VEGF treatment is self-financed, hindering access for the underprivileged. It has been mentioned that most public hospitals in the region are less likely to adopt a T&E regimen directly after the loading phase but are more inclined towards PRN regimen because of limited manpower and resources [7]. With the number of injections administered in the territory exponentially rising in recent years due to the ageing population, there is clearly a need to explore better alternatives to the PRN approach and this forms the basis of our study.

1.2. The Planned Quarterly Dosing after Three Loading Doses Regimen (QDA3L) Protocol

Generally, three monthly or four-weekly injections would be arranged for newly diagnosed patients with nAMD during the initial visit at our institution. Due to the difficulty of booking injections well in advance, some ophthalmologists would also help secure a further injection clinic booking at week 20 during that initial visit, on a case-by-case basis, primarily for operational reasons. No specific selection criteria were applied. These patients would be offered a follow-up appointment after the three loading doses, usually at week 12. The objective was to establish a consistent injection interval of 12 to 16 weeks. We have termed this regimen "planned quarterly dosing after three loading doses" (QDA3L) (Figure 1). Previous guidelines suggested that the interval between injections could be extended in four-week increments after the three initial doses, up to a maximum interval of 12 weeks for patients with inactive disease [8]. The ALTAIR study confirmed that a large proportion of patients (35.1–40.5%) had an intended injection interval of 16 weeks by week 52 in patients treated with aflibercept for treatment-naïve exudative AMD [9]. The PIER and EXCITE studies were earlier trials that examined the fixed dosing regimen for ranibizumab [10,11]. The PIER study was a controlled trial that randomized patients with subfoveal MNV to receive sham or ranibizumab monthly for three months, followed by quarterly treatment. The EXCITE study randomised subjects to three initial monthly doses of ranibizumab, followed by a quarterly fixed regimen of different dosing (0.3 mg or 0.5 mg) or monthly ranibizumab. In line with the overall approach of these regimens to ultimately achieve an intended injection interval of 12 to 16 weeks, some of our doctors would discuss with our patients and maintain a fixed quarterly injection interval to sustain disease inactivity. This would reduce the burden of frequent clinic visits when the patient is on a stable treatment protocol.

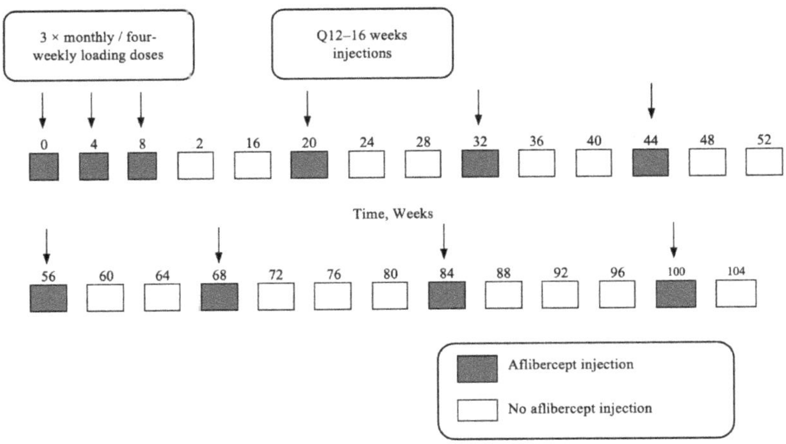

Figure 1. Example of a quarterly dosing after three loading doses (QDA3L) regimen.

During each clinic visit, patients underwent visual acuity (VA) testing, optical coherence tomography (OCT), slit lamp biomicroscopy, indirect ophthalmoscopy, and fundus photos for selected cases. During the week 12 appointment and subsequent appointments, the decision on whether to maintain the treatment interval would be made. If there were no signs of increase in activity, the injection at week 20 would be kept, and subsequent injection intervals would be between 12 and 16 weeks (Figure 1). Any decision to shorten the treatment interval to below 12 weeks, due to increased activity, would be regarded as failing the intended planned quarterly dosing.

2. Materials and Methods

2.1. Study Setting and Population

In light of the increasing treatment burden for all parties involved, we decided to look into whether some fixed, straightforward, and less-treatment intensive regimens would be comparable to the current widely practised treat-and-extend (T&E) regimen [12]. We aimed to investigate the success rate of a planned quarterly aflibercept injection schedule, following three initial loading doses of aflibercept, for neovascular age-related macular degeneration (nAMD) to achieve stability without recurrence at a tertiary eye centre. Our goal is to test the hypothesis that a less frequent dosing regimen may be sustainable to our healthcare system and beneficial to our patients, allowing for a stable disease state without recurrence while reducing the treatment burden and the frequency of visits to an acceptable level.

A retrospective study of electronic health records was conducted, including all consecutive cases of nAMD treated with three initial aflibercept injections four weeks apart, followed by a planned injection appointment at week 20 for at least one year, at United Christian Hospital and Tseung Kwan O Hospital in Hong Kong, over five years (January 2017–December 2021). Our centres provide tertiary eye care to the eastern peninsula of Kowloon in Hong Kong, China, with a catchment population of 1.1 million.

The study received approval from the local research ethics committee (Reference: KC/KE-23-0029/ER-3) and complied with the Declaration of Helsinki.

2.2. Inclusion and Exclusion Criteria

Inclusion and exclusion criteria were adopted from major randomized controlled trials (RCTs) [4,9]. The inclusion criteria were as follows: subjects aged over 50 years, neovascular AMD with foveal involvement, both treatment-naïve and recurrent cases, and patients who had injections for at least one year. There were no specific criteria for initial best-correted visual acuity (BCVA). Only active subfoveal MNV were included, including types 1, 2, and 3. Polypoidal choroidal vasculopathy (PCV), a variant of type 1 MNV, was included to represent the real-life data in our locality.

Exclusion criteria were as follows: eyes that received any anti-VEGF therapy in the prior six months, eyes with other disease entities (e.g., diabetic macula oedema, retinal vein occlusions, central serous chorioretinopathy, myopic macular neovascularisation), a follow-up period of less than one year, concurrent macula laser (except photodynamic therapy) and ocular surgery (e.g., cataract surgery or vitrectomy) in the prior six months and the study period, planned injections between week 12 and week 19, and patients who decided to stop injections and opted for a PRN regimen after three injections or within the first year.

2.3. Imaging and Evaluation

The spectral-domain optical coherence tomography (SD-OCT) (Spectralis, Heidelberg Engineering, Heidelberg, Germany), fundus fluorescein angiography (FFA), and indocyanine green angiography (ICGA) (Spectralis HRA+OCT, Heidelberg Engineering, Heidelberg, Germany) images were reviewed. In this retrospective study, the neovascular lesions were classified and confirmed via the reviewing of all the multimodal imaging available for each case by one retinal specialist. The subtypes of nAMD were classified according to FFA, ICGA, and OCT findings. Subjects were confirmed to have nAMD with foveal involvement, with confirmation of leakage on fundus fluorescein angiogram before the start of treatment. All cases of PCV were confirmed with ICGA [13]. OCT was the primary imaging modality used to assess dryness of the fovea. Safety evaluation was recorded in clinical notes if any positive findings were observed. Major adverse events screened for included endophthalmitis, retinal detachment, hyphema, vitreous haemorrhage, retinal pigment epithelium tear, thromboembolic events, and death related to the injection.

2.4. Treatment Success and Failure

Our definitions of treatment success include overall, anatomical, and functional at W52 and W104. Anatomical success was defined as no increase in disease activity of the AMD on clinical examination or OCT throughout the study period while remaining on the quarterly dosing schedule, without the need to shorten the treatment interval. Functional success was characterised by a loss of fewer than five ETDRS letters, without the need to shorten the treatment interval. Overall success combined both. Treatment failure was defined as an increase in disease activity during the two-year quarterly dosing maintenance stage, i.e. new macular haemorrhage, neovascularisation, and/or an increase in OCT biomarkers for neovascular activity, and thus a decision for rescue treatment with shorter treatment intervals. The widely recognized OCT biomarkers for neovascular activity, including intraretinal fluid, subretinal fluid, subretinal pigment epithelium fluid, and subretinal hyperreflective material, were used when supplementing the clinical findings with OCT response [14–17].

2.5. Statistical Analysis

Frequencies were compared between the groups using either chi-square test or Fisher's exact test. Continuous unpaired data were compared using Mann–Whitney U test and change in visual acuity with Friedman test and Kruskal–Wallis test. Success rates and outcomes were summarised descriptively. The two-sided 95% confidence intervals of the proportions of success and failure were estimated using normal approximation. A p value of less than 0.05 was considered statistically significant. Statistical evaluation was performed using SPSS software version 26 (IBM, Armonk, NY, USA).

3. Results

The flow diagram showing subject recruitment is shown in Figure 2 and the patient demographics are summarised in Table 1. A total of 956 eyes met the criteria of nAMD requiring anti-VEGF in the 5-year study period. Among these, 57 eyes met the inclusion criteria for following the QDA3L schedule with aflibercept. However, 17 of them were excluded due to various reasons, such as not having completed at least one year of injections, voluntary withdrawal, receiving anti-VEGF in the 6 months prior to the study, and undergoing intraocular surgery (Table 2). Of the remaining 40 eyes of 40 patients, 18 cases had polypoidal choroidal vasculopathy (PCV); 6 of them had concurrent photodynamic therapy (PDT) within the first month of their first injection, and thus they were excluded from the main monotherapy group analysis. These six eyes in the combination therapy group were analysed separately. None of the included PCV cases received PDT outside the first month period throughout the study.

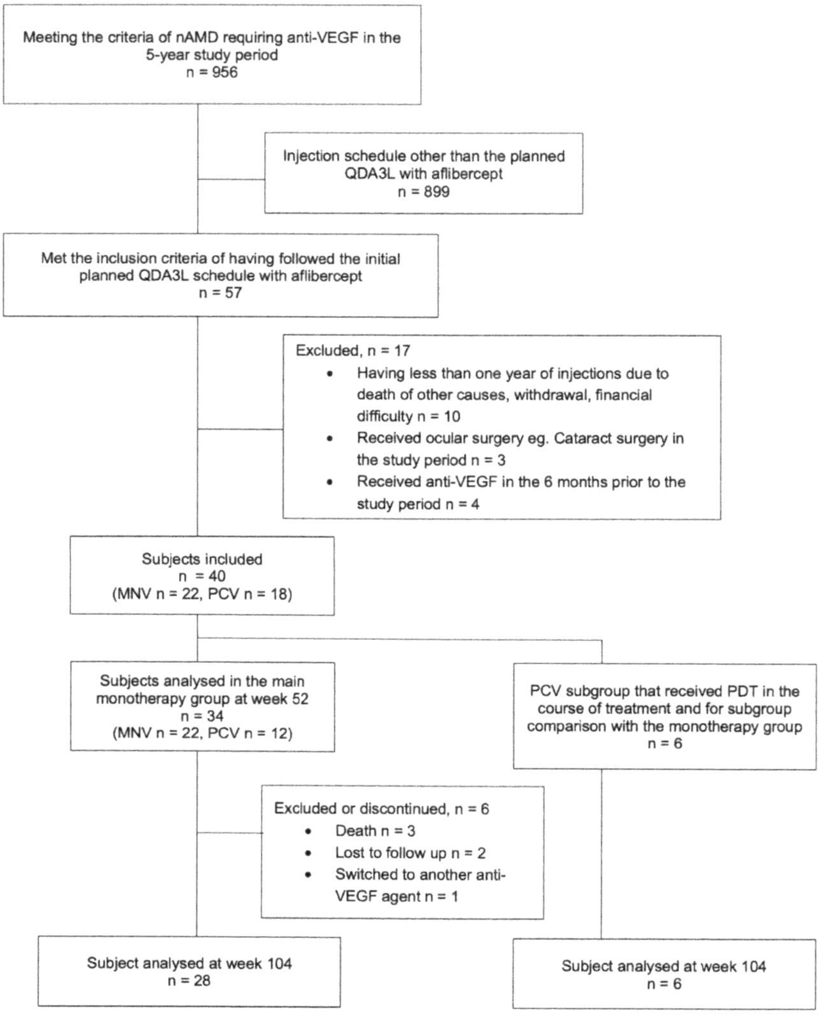

Figure 2. Flow diagram showing the number of patients assessed for eligibility, included in the study, and analysed at each time point. nAMD: neovascular age-related macular degeneration. QDA3L: quarterly dosing after three loading doses. MNV: macular neovascularization. PCV: polypoidal choroidal vasculopathy. PDT: photodynamic therapy. Anti-VEGF: anti-vascular endothelial growth factor.

A total of 34 eyes of 34 patients were included in the aflibercept monotherapy group and analysed. Among them, 24 cases were treatment-naïve, and 10 were recurrence cases. In total, 64.7% (n = 22) of them had a diagnosis of macular neovascularisation (MNV), and 12 of them had PCV with monotherapy. Among the MNV group, 59% (n = 13) had type 1 MNV, 36% (n = 8) had type 2 MNV, and one case had type 3 MNV.

Table 1. Patient demographics of the main monotherapy group.

	n = 34 (%)	p Value for Treatment Success at 1 Year
Age		0.85 #
• Mean ± SD	80.8 ± 7.9	
• Median (min–max)	81 (64–97)	
Laterality, n (% left)	13 (38.2%)	0.62 ^
Gender, n (% female)	12 (35.2%)	0.47 ^
Ethnicity		
• Chinese	40 (100%)	
Diagnosis		0.22 ^
• MNV	22 (64.7%)	
○ Type 1 MNV	13	
○ Type 2 MNV	8	
○ Type 3 MNV	1	
• PCV	12 (29.4%)	
Baseline visual acuity (ETDRS letters)		0.80 #
• Mean ± SD	46.93 ± 14.98	
• Median (min–max)	46.93 (19.95–73.91)	
Treatment more than 6 months before the first injection in the study period		0.27 ^
• Treatment-naïve	24 (70.5%)	
• Recurrence	10 (29.4%)	
Lens status		0.68 ^
• Pseudophakic	19 (55.9%)	
• Clear lens	1 (0.03%)	
• Nucleus sclerosis grade 1–2	14 (41.1%)	
• Nucleus sclerosis grade 3 or above	0	
Other ocular pathology		
• Nil	30 (88.2%)	-
• Epiretinal membrane	2 (0.05%)	-
• Old branch retinal vein occlusion	1 (0.03%)	-
• Normal tension glaucoma	1 (0.03%)	-

^ Chi-square or Fisher's exact test. # Mann–Whitney U test. SD: standard deviation. MNV: macular neovascularisation. ETDRS: Early Treatment of Diabetic Retinopathy Study.

Table 2. Excluded cases that initially met the quarterly dosing after three loading doses (QDA3L) schedule.

Reasons	n = 17
Having less than one year of injections (death of other causes, withdrawal, financial difficulty)	10
Having ocular surgery e.g., cataract surgery in the study period	3
Received anti-VEGF in the 6 months prior to the study period	4

Anti-VEGF: anti-vascular endothelial growth factor.

All patients underwent OCT imaging at their initial visit and subsequent visits. All patients had FFA before their first injection. All PCV cases had ICGA for diagnosis confirmation before their first injection. Not all MNV cases, however, had ICGA: 27% (n = 6) only had FFA.

The mean baseline visual acuity was 46.93 ± 14.98 letters. 55.9% (n = 19) of the cases were pseudophakic, and the rest had clear lens or mild cataract. A total of 88.2% of the cases did not have any co-existing macula pathology or glaucoma. Four of the cases had mild co-existing pathology such as epiretinal membrane or old retinal vein occlusion. All these did not show any statistical significance in relation to treatment success or failure.

The mean visual acuity across the subjects improved with treatment, and the final visual outcomes are summarised in Table 3. The overall anatomical and functional success at W52 and W104 in our cohort are summarised in Table 4. The mean change in BCVA (ETDRS letters) after three loading doses, from baseline to week 52, and from baseline to week 104 was 5.4 letters (95% CI −0.6 to 11.4), 3.5 letters (95% CI −3.7 to 10.6), and 1.7 letters, respectively (95% CI −4.3 to 7.7). The proportion of subjects who achieved anatomical success at week 52 and week 104 was 73.5% (95% CI 58.7% to 88.4%) and 64.3% (95% CI 46.5% to 82.0%), respectively. The proportion of subjects who achieved functional success at week 52 and week 104 was 55.8% (95% CI 39.2% to 75.6%) and 53.6% (95% CI 35.1% to 72.0%), respectively. The overall success rate in our study population was 52.9% (95% CI 36.2% to 69.7%) at week 52 and 53.6% (95% CI 35.1% to 72.0%) at week 104. The anatomical success rate was higher than the corresponding functional success rate. There were no major adverse events reported during the study period.

Table 3. Functional outcomes.

	ETDRS Score	p-Value #
Baseline visual acuity		
• Mean ± SD	46.93 ± 14.98	-
• Median (min–max)	46.93 (19.95–73.91)	
Visual acuity after first 3 injections		
• Mean ± SD	52.35 ± 17.81	0.01 [a] @
• Median (min, max)	58.86 (6.57–80.15)	
Visual acuity at Week 52		
• Mean ± SD	50.37 ± 21.11	0.15 [a] 0.26 [b]
• Median (min, max)	54.45 (19.95–82.71)	
Visual acuity at Week 104 ^		
• Mean ± SD	45.90 ± 22.70	0.47 [a] 0.06 [b] 0.47 [c]
• Median (min, max)	46.93 (6.57–77.25)	

Friedman test with post hoc analysis. [a] vs. baseline. [b] vs. after three injections. [c] vs. week 52. @ $p < 0.05$. ^ Only cases who had follow-up at week 104 (2 years) and who were not excluded from the study were analysed ($n = 28$). ETDRS: Early Treatment of Diabetic Retinopathy Study. SD: Standard deviation.

Table 4. Overall, anatomical, and functional success at W52 and W104 in our cohort.

		Anatomical Success #	Functional Success #	Overall Success
Week 52	n	25/34	19/34	18/34
	% (95% CI)	73.5% (58.7% to 88.4%)	55.8% (39.2% to 75.6%)	52.9% (36.2% to 69.7%)
Week 104 ^	n	18/28	15/28	15/28
	% (95% CI)	64.3% (46.5% to 82.0%)	53.6% (35.1% to 72.0%)	53.6% (35.1% to 72.0%)

Anatomical success was defined as no increase in activity of the AMD on clinical examination and OCT throughout the study period without the need to shorten the treatment interval. Functional success was characterised by a loss of fewer than five ETDRS letters without the need to shorten the treatment interval. Overall success combined both. ^ 6 were excluded from analysis for functional success at week 104, yielding only 28 cases for analyses, due to the following events after 1 year: death ($n = 3$), lost to follow-up ($n = 2$), switched to another anti-VEGF agent ($n = 1$). 95% CI: 95% confidence interval.

Regardless of the anatomical success during the study period, the fovea remained dry on OCT in 85.3% ($n = 29/34$, 95% CI 73.4% to 97.2%) and 82.1% ($n = 23/28$, 95% CI 68.0% to 96.3%) of the cases at week 52 and week 104, respectively. The proportion of subjects who lost fewer than 15 ETDRS letters was 85.3% (95% CI 73.4% to 97.2%) and 85.7% (95% CI 72.8% to 98.7%) at weeks 52 and 104, respectively. The proportion of subjects who gained more than 15 ETDRS letters was 35.3% (95% CI 19.2% to 51.4%) and 25.0% (95% CI 9.0% to 41.0%) at weeks 52 and 104, respectively.

The visual acuity after the initial loading doses, but not the VA at weeks 52 or 104, showed a significant difference from with the baseline VA (Friedman test, $p = 0.01$) (Table 3). Between the treatment success and failure groups, there was no statistical difference in the baseline demographics, including gender, age at presentation, baseline visual acuity, whether treatment-naïve or recurrent cases, and lens status. The survival curve is shown in Figure 3. Subgroup analysis for treatment outcomes is shown in Table 5. Statistical analysis did not show a significant difference in outcomes among the different groups of MNV (Table 6). Comparison of outcomes was also performed between the aflibercept monotherapy group and the combination treatment group with PDT for the PCV cases, and the results are shown in Table 7. Due to the small sample size of the PDT subgroup, no significant conclusion can be drawn, although both groups had a fair success rate.

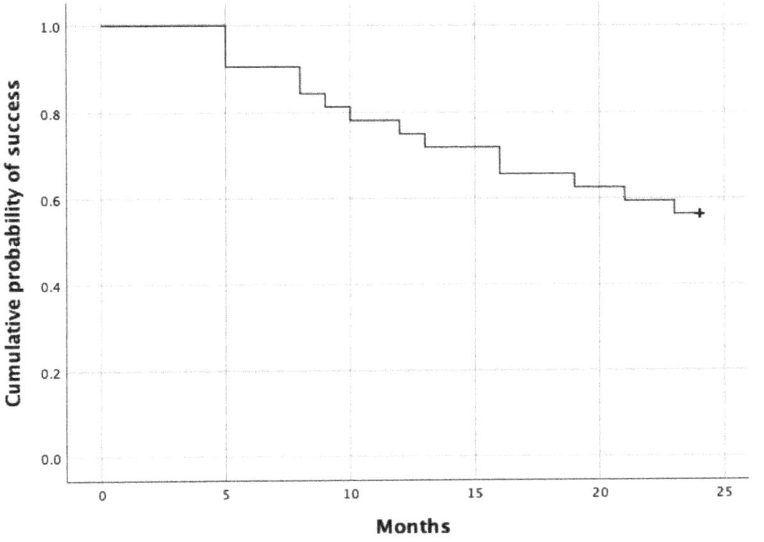

Figure 3. Kaplan–Meier survival curve for treatment to failure time (in months) in our cohort.

Table 5. Subgroup analysis of the overall, anatomical, and functional success at week 52 and week 104 for type 1 and type 2 MNV and PCV monotherapy.

	Anatomical Success	Functional Success	Overall Success
Type 1 MNV—Week 52	10/13 (76.9%)	8/13 (61.5%)	7/13 (53.8%)
Type 2 MNV—Week 52	6/8 (75.0%)	4/8 (50.0%)	4/8 (50.0%)
PCV monotherapy—Week 52	9/12 (75.0%)	7/12 (58.3%)	7/12 (58.3%)
Type 1 MNV—Week 104 ^a	5/10 (50.0%)	5/10 (50.0%)	5/10 (50.0%)
Type 2 MNV— Week 104 ^b	5/7 (71.4%)	3/7 (42.9%)	3/7 (42.9%)
PCV monotherapy—Week 104 ^c	8/11 (72.7%)	7/11 (63.6%)	7/11 (63.6%)

^a Excluded as subjects passed away $n = 2$ and was lost to follow up $n = 1$. ^b Excluded as subject was lost to follow up $n = 1$. ^c Excluded as subject passed away after week 52 $n = 1$. MNV: macular neovascularisation. PCV: polypoidal choroidal vasculopathy.

Table 6. Subgroup comparison of outcomes for type 1 MNV, type 2 MNV, and PCV monotherapy (p-value).

	After 3 Injections	Week 52	Week 104
Visual acuity gain #	0.49	0.42	0.55
Anatomical success ^	-	0.50	0.87
Functional success ^	-	0.87	0.66
Overall success ^	-	0.93	0.66
Dryness of fovea ^	-	0.86	0.33

Kruskal–Wallis test. ^ Chi-square test. MNV: macular neovascularisation. PCV: polypoidal choroidal vasculopathy.

Table 7. Subgroup analysis of the combo and anti-VEGF monotherapy group of polypoidal choroidal vasculopathy on the overall, anatomical, and functional success at W52 and W104.

	Anatomical Success	Functional Success	Overall Success
Monotherapy—Week 52	9/12 (75.0%)	7/12 (58.3%)	7/12 (58.3%)
Combination therapy—Week 52	5/6 (83.3%)	5/6 (83.3%)	5/6 (83.3%)
Monotherapy—Week 104 ^	8/11 (72.7%)	7/11 (63.6%)	7/11 (63.6%)
Combination therapy—Week 104 ^	4/6 (66.7%)	4/6 (66.7%)	4/6 (66.7%)

^ Excluded at 104 as subject passed away after week 52 n = 1. Anti-VEGF: anti-vascular endothelial growth factor.

4. Discussion

Hong Kong is a densely populated city, and many people in our locality still live in poverty. Although subsidized programmes from the government and charitable programmes from private organisations are available in limited numbers, treating macular disease with anti-VEGF has been an enormous burden to our ophthalmic services. As these injections are locally self-financed, patients who are experiencing financial pressure in our locality cannot afford or are unwilling to comply with tight injection schedules. This group of patients opt out of the treat-and-extend regimen and prefer a pro re nata (PRN) approach instead.

In 2020, a panel of retinal experts from the United Kingdom released practical guidance and recommendations to optimize the aflibercept T&E pathway for nAMD patients that could be implemented in clinical practice [12]. They recommended, for aflibercept, an initial loading phase with three injections four weeks apart, followed by the fourth injection at week 20, and then a decision as to whether to maintain injections every eight weeks or to extend the injection interval by 2 to 4 weeks for active and inactive disease, respectively. The incremental intervals were set at two to four weeks.

Quarterly dosing was studied in larger, multicentre, randomised controlled trials [18]. Both the PIER and EXCITE studies, which were published over a decade ago, studied ranibizumab and found quarterly dosing inferior to monthly dosing [10,11]. There has been a lack of similar studies on fixed quarterly dosing for aflibercept in the past decade. Studies have shown that the intraocular suppression times of VEGF following intravitreal aflibercept in human eyes can last up to 16 weeks [9,19]. Therefore, dosing every 12 to 16 weeks could theoretically be useful to suppress VEGF to prevent recurrence. The subsequent landmark studies, such as ALTAIR, on aflibercept dosing of intervals longer than their labelled bimonthly dosing, were based on a stepwise T&E increment to a 16-week interval [20]. Khanna et al. commented that the switch of research focus to variable frequency anti-VEGF regimens resulted from the unfavourable outcomes from PIER and EXCITE [18]. Subjects in the PIER study were monitored and treated quarterly [18].

Compared to the traditional treat and extend regimen, by planning the fourth injection at week 20, the injection interval will be extended all the way to 12–16 weeks in the QDA3L regimen, without incremental intervals of 2 to 4 weeks. In our study, those who demonstrated increased activity were considered treatment failures and received earlier rescue injections. In prospective real-life practice, we recommend closer monthly follow-up during the initial 'extend' period between week 8 and week 20, prior to the injection at week 20. This allows for some degree of individualisation to prevent undertreatment and to identify cases that are stable enough and approaching a dry fovea before transitioning to the QDA3L schedule.

In the ALTAIR study published in 2019, 246 patients were randomised at week 16, after three initial doses of aflibercept, 1:1 to T&E with either 2- or 4-week adjustments [9]. This study was the first randomised controlled study to examine the outcomes associated with 4-week adjustments and injection intervals beyond 12 weeks for aflibercept-treated patients [9]. The proportion of subjects with the last injection interval of 12 weeks or longer was 43.2–49.6% for both groups up to week 52 and 56.9–60.2% up to week 96 [9]. The

AIRES study in 2021 was a randomized study involving 271 patients having received aflibercept. Their regimen involved monthly injections till week 16, after which patients were randomised into early-start (with 2-week interval adjustments) or late-start (8-week intervals until W48 then 2-week interval adjustments) T&E [4]. The percentage of patients with the last treatment intervals of 12 weeks or longer up to week 104 was between 47.2 and 51.9% for the early start T&E and late-start T&E groups, respectively [4]. Due to the retrospective nature of our study, while we are not able to compare head-to-head with the randomised trials, our initial study result shows that our protocol has a fair and acceptable response to this group of patients. It should also be noted that our population had a worse baseline visual acuity before treatment and a higher proportion of patients with PCV.

Our study is based on real-life patient data and is not a large randomised clinical trial like ALTAIR or AIRES. In our public healthcare setting, there is a waiting time between the initial visit date and the first injection. Nevertheless, we acknowledge certain weaknesses in the present study, including its retrospective nature and small sample size. The selection of patients into this quarterly regimen by individual doctors at the clinic could result in selection bias, although we did not observe any specific patient population that would be favoured for selection for this booking of the initial four injections at the initial visit, other than for operational reasons. The strict inclusion criteria also mean that this only represented a small proportion of all the injections performed at our institution in the study period. Recent evidence also suggested the use of optical coherence tomography angiography (OCT-A) as a non-invasive technique for detecting macular neovascularisation cases with persistent fluid [14]. We acknowledge the lack of use of such imaging modality in our cases during the study period. Furthermore, it should be noted that our results may not be generalisable to other populations worldwide as all cases in our study were of Chinese ethnicity. Further prospective controlled trials with larger sample size, detailed rescue criteria, and investigations into the success rate of anti-VEGF treatment for different types of MNV may provide additional evidence to support our conclusions.

5. Conclusions

Quarterly aflibercept injections after three initial doses were able to maintain a dry fovea for 82.1 to 85.3% of the patients in our locality; 85.3% to 85.7% of patients lost fewer than 15 ETDRS letters, with an overall success rate of 52.9% at 1 year and 53.6% at 2 years. This regimen can be recommended to patients in our locality who have financial constraints and prefer an alternative to the PRN approach, with a lower number of injections. It is important to note that various treatment regimens have been described in the literature, and this retrospective study does not imply the superiority or inferiority of this regimen. Further prospective controlled trials of larger sample sizes may provide more evidence for our conclusions. The success and failure rates observed in our study can provide information for counselling patients considering this specific fixed treatment regimen.

Author Contributions: Conceptualization, D.H.T.W. and K.K.W.L.; methodology, D.H.T.W.; formal analysis, D.H.T.W.; data curation, D.H.T.W.; writing—original draft preparation, D.H.T.W.; writing—review and editing, D.H.T.W. and K.K.W.L.; supervision, K.K.W.L. All authors have read and agreed to the published version of the manuscript.

Funding: This research received no external funding.

Institutional Review Board Statement: The study was conducted in accordance with the Declaration of Helsinki and approved by the Research Ethics Committee (Kowloon Central/ Kowloon East) of Hospital Authority, Hong Kong SAR, China (Reference: KC/KE-23-0029/ER-3 and date of approval 1 August 2023).

Informed Consent Statement: Patient consent was waived due to the retrospective nature of this study.

Data Availability Statement: The anonymized data presented in this study are available on request from the corresponding author. The data are not publicly available due to patient confidentially.

Acknowledgments: The authors would like to acknowledge Jeremy Tsang for his help with statistical analysis.

Conflicts of Interest: The authors declare no conflicts of interest.

References

1. Wong, W.L.; Su, X.; Li, X.; Cheung, C.M.; Klein, R.; Cheng, C.Y.; Wong, T.Y. Global prevalence of age-related macular degeneration and disease burden projection for 2020 and 2040: A systematic review and meta-analysis. *Lancet Glob. Health* **2014**, *2*, e106–e116. [CrossRef] [PubMed]
2. Ambati, J.; Fowler, B.J. Mechanisms of age-related macular degeneration. *Neuron* **2012**, *75*, 26–39. [CrossRef] [PubMed]
3. Lanzetta, P.; Loewenstein, A.; Vision Academy Steering Committee. Fundamental principles of an anti-VEGF treatment regimen: Optimal application of intravitreal anti-vascular endothelial growth factor therapy of macular diseases. *Graefes Arch. Clin. Exp. Ophthalmol.* **2017**, *255*, 1259–1273. [CrossRef] [PubMed]
4. Mitchell, P.; Holz, F.G.; Hykin, P.; Midena, E.; Souied, E.; Allmeier, H.; Lambrou, G.; Schmelter, T.; Wolf, S. Efficacy and Safety of Intravitreal Aflibercept Using a Treat-and-Extend Regimen for Neovascular Age-Related Macular Degeneration: The ARIES Study: A Randomized Clinical Trial. *Retina* **2021**, *41*, 1911–1920. [CrossRef] [PubMed]
5. Comparison of Age-related Macular Degeneration Treatments Trials Research Group; Maguire, M.G.; Martin, D.F.; Ying, G.S.; Jaffe, G.J.; Daniel, E.; Grunwald, J.E.; Toth, C.A.; Ferris, F.L., 3rd; Fine, S.L. Five-Year Outcomes with Anti-Vascular Endothelial Growth Factor Treatment of Neovascular Age-Related Macular Degeneration: The Comparison of Age-Related Macular Degeneration Treatments Trials. *Ophthalmology* **2016**, *123*, 1751–1761. [CrossRef] [PubMed]
6. Reitan, G.; Kjellevold Haugen, I.B.; Andersen, K.; Bragadottir, R.; Bindesboll, C. Through the Eyes of Patients: Understanding Treatment Burden of Intravitreal Anti-VEGF Injections for nAMD Patients in Norway. *Clin. Ophthalmol.* **2023**, *17*, 1465–1474. [CrossRef] [PubMed]
7. Kwok, A.K.; Lam, W.C.; Fong, A.H.; Fung, N.S.; Ho, M.; Iu, L.P.; Ko, C.; Mohamed, S.; Ng, D.; Tang, H.; et al. Recommendations of the treat-and-extend regimen for neovascular age-related macular degeneration: 2020 updates. *Hong Kong J. Ophthalmol.* **2021**, *25*, 39–46. [CrossRef]
8. Koh, A.; Lanzetta, P.; Lee, W.K.; Lai, C.C.; Chan, W.M.; Yang, C.M.; Cheung, C.M. Recommended Guidelines for Use of Intravitreal Aflibercept with a Treat-and-Extend Regimen for the Management of Neovascular Age-Related Macular Degeneration in the Asia-Pacific Region: Report from a Consensus Panel. *Asia-Pac. J. Ophthalmol.* **2017**, *6*, 296–302.
9. Ohji, M.; Takahashi, K.; Okada, A.A.; Kobayashi, M.; Matsuda, Y.; Terano, Y. Efficacy and Safety of Intravitreal Aflibercept Treat-and-Extend Regimens in Exudative Age-Related Macular Degeneration: 52- and 96-Week Findings from ALTAIR: A Randomized Controlled Trial. *Adv. Ther.* **2020**, *37*, 1173–1187. [CrossRef] [PubMed]
10. Abraham, P.; Yue, H.; Wilson, L. Randomized, double-masked, sham-controlled trial of ranibizumab for neovascular age-related macular degeneration: PIER study year 2. *Am. J. Ophthalmol.* **2010**, *150*, 315–324.e1. [CrossRef] [PubMed]
11. Schmidt-Erfurth, U.; Eldem, B.; Guymer, R.; Korobelnik, J.F.; Schlingemann, R.O.; Axer-Siegel, R.; Wiedemann, P.; Simader, C.; Gekkieva, M.; Weichselberger, A.; et al. Efficacy and safety of monthly versus quarterly ranibizumab treatment in neovascular age-related macular degeneration: The EXCITE study. *Ophthalmology* **2011**, *118*, 831–839. [CrossRef] [PubMed]
12. Ross, A.H.; Downey, L.; Devonport, H.; Gale, R.P.; Kotagiri, A.; Mahmood, S.; Mehta, H.; Narendran, N.; Patel, P.J.; Parmar, N.; et al. Recommendations by a UK expert panel on an aflibercept treat-and-extend pathway for the treatment of neovascular age-related macular degeneration. *Eye* **2020**, *34*, 1825–1834. [CrossRef] [PubMed]
13. Lee, W.K.; Iida, T.; Ogura, Y.; Chen, S.J.; Wong, T.Y.; Mitchell, P.; Cheung, G.C.M.; Zhang, Z.; Leal, S.; Ishibashi, T.; et al. Efficacy and Safety of Intravitreal Aflibercept for Polypoidal Choroidal Vasculopathy in the PLANET Study: A Randomized Clinical Trial. *JAMA Ophthalmol.* **2018**, *136*, 786–793. [CrossRef] [PubMed]
14. Fouad, Y.A.; Santina, A.; Bousquet, E.; Sadda, S.R.; Sarraf, D. Pathways of Fluid Leakage in Age Related Macular Degeneration. *Retina* **2023**, *43*, 873–881. [CrossRef] [PubMed]
15. Wong, D.T.; Berger, A.R.; Bourgault, S.; Chen, J.; Colleaux, K.; Cruess, A.F.; Dookeran, R.I.; Gauthier, D.; Hurley, B.; Kapusta, M.A.; et al. Imaging Biomarkers and Their Impact on Therapeutic Decision-Making in the Management of Neovascular Age-Related Macular Degeneration. *Ophthalmologica* **2021**, *244*, 265–280. [CrossRef] [PubMed]
16. Schmidt-Erfurth, U.; Waldstein, S.M. A paradigm shift in imaging biomarkers in neovascular age-related macular degeneration. *Prog. Retin. Eye Res.* **2016**, *50*, 1–24. [CrossRef] [PubMed]
17. Holekamp, N.M.; Sadda, S.; Sarraf, D.; Guymer, R.; Hill, L.; Blotner, S.; Spicer, G.; Gune, S. Effect of Residual Retinal Fluid on Visual Function in Ranibizumab-Treated Neovascular Age-Related Macular Degeneration. *Am. J. Ophthalmol.* **2022**, *233*, 8–17. [CrossRef] [PubMed]

18. Khanna, S.; Komati, R.; Eichenbaum, D.A.; Hariprasad, I.; Ciulla, T.A.; Hariprasad, S.M. Current and upcoming anti-VEGF therapies and dosing strategies for the treatment of neovascular AMD: A comparative review. *BMJ Open Ophthalmol.* **2019**, *4*, e000398. [CrossRef] [PubMed]
19. Fauser, S.; Schwabecker, V.; Muether, P.S. Suppression of intraocular vascular endothelial growth factor during aflibercept treatment of age-related macular degeneration. *Am. J. Ophthalmol.* **2014**, *158*, 532–536. [CrossRef] [PubMed]
20. Anguita, R.; Tasiopoulou, A.; Shahid, S.; Roth, J.; Sim, S.Y.; Patel, P.J. A Review of Aflibercept Treatment for Macular Disease. *Ophthalmol. Ther.* **2021**, *10*, 413–428. [CrossRef] [PubMed]

Journal of
Clinical Medicine

MDPI

Systematic Review

COVID-19 Related Retinal Vascular Occlusion: A Systematic Review

Argyrios Tzamalis *, Maria Foti, Maria Georgiadou, Nikolaos Tsaftaridis and Nikolaos Ziakas

2nd Department of Ophthalmology, Aristotle University of Thessaloniki, Papageorgiou General Hospital, 564 29 Thessaloniki, Greece; mariafoti@auth.gr (M.F.); mtgeorgiad@gmail.com (M.G.); tsaftaridis1@gmail.com (N.T.); nikolasziakas@gmail.com (N.Z.)

* Correspondence: argyriostzamalis@yahoo.com; Tel.: +30-6942060467; Fax: +30-2313323974

Abstract: Background/Objectives: To provide insight into populations at higher risk of COVID-19-related retinal vascular occlusion, we identified the baseline characteristics of COVID-19 patients and vaccine recipients who developed this condition by conducting a systematic review to summarize the findings and evaluate the current knowledge on this subject. **Methods**: An electronic search on the PubMed and Scopus databases was performed for relevant case reports or series regarding retinal vascular occlusion in patients with past or present COVID-19 infection or SARS-CoV-2 immunization. This study was conducted using a pre-determined protocol following the Preferred Reporting Items for Systematic Reviews and Meta-Analyses (PRISMA) guidelines. **Results**: A total of 34 studies were enrolled in this systematic review. A total of 21 patients (14 males, 66.7%) have been diagnosed with COVID-19 related retinal vein occlusion (RVO, mean age = 41.9 $\pm$ 10.3 years), and 15 patients (12 males, 80%) have been diagnosed with retinal artery occlusion (RAO, mean age = 56.9 $\pm$ 13.2 years). The time to RVO since COVID-19 infection or SARS-CoV-2 immunization ranged from 8 h to 51 days (mean = 12.3 $\pm$ 15.7 days), while the time to RAO ranged from 2 to 40 days (mean = 14.9 $\pm$ 10.8 days). Fifteen out of the twenty-one patients (71.4%) with RVO had a significant improvement in visual acuity after the resolution of symptoms while eight out of the fifteen patients (53.3%) with RAO did not show improvement. **Conclusions**: COVID-19 seems to play a significant role in the pathogenesis of vascular occlusion, as it is suggested to increase the risk of thromboembolic episodes. However, the pathophysiologic mechanisms have not been fully elucidated, and further studies are expected to shed light on this phenomenon.

Keywords: COVID-19; SARS-CoV-2; vaccination; retinal vascular occlusion; vein occlusion; artery occlusion

1. Introduction

Although COVID-19 affects mainly the respiratory system, it has also been associated with coagulopathies and venous or arterial thromboembolism [1,2]. Moreover, SARS-CoV-2 infection is associated with ocular manifestations, such as conjunctivitis (most common), changes in the retinal vasculature, and ocular thromboembolic events [3].

Retinal vascular occlusions are divided into two main categories: Retinal vein occlusions (RVO) and retinal artery occlusions (RAO), the former being much more common than the latter, with a better prognosis. Common risk factors for both types of occlusions are age over 50 years and the presence of cardiovascular risk factors [4]. Most acute artery occlusions are embolic, secondary to internal carotid artery disease. Non-embolic occlusions can occur from vasculitis and infectious causes. On the other side, predisposing factors for retinal vein thrombosis are hypertension, diabetes, arterial nicking (narrowing), and glaucoma [5].

The first case of ocular vascular occlusion (OVO) related to COVID-19 infection was published only some months after the pandemic outbreak, in June 2020 [6], while the first case of OVO related to COVID-19 vaccination was reported in January 2022 [7], and soon additional, similar case reports started emerging [8–39]. Although several cases have already been published on this subject, there is still controversy regarding the true relationship between COVID-19 and retinal vascular occlusion events. Therefore, we have conducted a systematic review attempting to summarize the findings and evaluate the current knowledge on this topic.

The primary objective of this study was to identify the baseline characteristics of COVID-19 patients and vaccine recipients who are more likely to develop retinal vascular occlusion, attempting to provide insight into populations at higher risk. The secondary objective was to thoroughly review these cases' presenting clinical images, laboratory examinations, management strategies, and outcomes, attempting to evaluate the association between COVID-19 and retinal vascular occlusion.

2. Methods

2.1. Conduct of Review

This study was conducted in line with a pre-determined protocol agreed upon by all co-authors, following the Preferred Reporting Items for Systematic Reviews and Meta-Analyses (PRISMA) guidelines.

2.2. Search Strategy and Study Selection

An electronic search on the PubMed and Scopus databases was performed (end date 3 November 2024) for relevant case reports or case series regarding retinal vascular occlusion in patients with past or present COVID-19 infection or SARS-CoV-2 immunization. The search terms used are thoroughly presented in Figure 1. Time restrictions were applied from 2019 to that date, and no linguistic restrictions were used. Subsequently, all relevant articles were screened for eligibility against the inclusion/exclusion criteria by three independent reviewers (NT, MG, MF). Articles were included if they involved patients with a history of COVID-19 infection or SARS-CoV-2 immunization and if they reported on retinal vascular occlusion in those patients. Articles were excluded if they did not present original data, had incomplete data, or did not meet certain additional eligibility criteria. These criteria encompassed articles not available in English, reporting on booster vaccinations, involving patients under 16 years old, and articles without confirmed COVID-19 infection or vaccination before or at the onset of ocular symptoms. Additional exclusions were applied for articles involving conditions beyond COVID-19 and retinal vascular occlusion, for articles with combined retinal vascular occlusion, and for articles where an additional COVID-19 infection or vaccination occurred after the retinal vascular occlusion, as these could confound the results. Finally, the three independent reviewers systematically reviewed the reference lists of eligible manuscripts ("snowballing") for potentially eligible articles. The search aimed to find original articles describing retinal vascular occlusion in COVID-19 patients or vaccine recipients. For this reason, review articles and correspondence presenting original data were included. Institutional review board approval was obtained before data extraction. The research methodology complied with the principles of the Declaration of Helsinki. The requirement for informed consent was waived due to the retrospective nature of the study.

PubMed search terms:

(COVID-19 OR covid-19 OR SARS-CoV-2 OR COVID-19 vaccine* "COVID-19"[Mesh] OR "SARS-CoV-2"[Mesh] OR "COVID-19 Vaccines"[Mesh]) AND ((retina* AND (vascular OR vessel OR vein* OR arter* OR papillophlebitis)) AND (occlusion OR thromb*)) OR ("Retinal Vein Occlusion"[Mesh] OR "Retinal Artery Occlusion"[Mesh])

Scopus search terms:

(Covid-19 OR SARS-CoV-2 OR (covid-19 AND vaccine)) AND ((retinal AND (vascular OR vein OR artery)) AND (occlusion OR thrombosis))

Figure 1. Search terms used for conducting this systematic review.

2.3. Data Extraction

The articles included in the study were reviewed by three independent reviewers. Data were extracted and organized into a pre-piloted, standardized form. Each reviewer independently extracted the data, and any discrepancies identified were resolved through consensus, with input from a senior author (AT). We identified and extracted the following data for analysis from each paper, where available: number of patients, age, weight, BMI, sex, comorbidities, type of ophthalmic vascular occlusion, occlusion symptoms, vaccine type, method of COVID-19 diagnosis, laboratory exams, previous COVID-19 diagnosis status, relevant imaging studies, exam findings, clinical features, management, and outcome.

2.4. Statistical Analysis

Statistical analysis was performed with Medcalc statistical software (version 9.3.0.0, Medcalc, Mariakerke, Belgium) and SPSS (v. 22.0 for Windows, SPSS INC, Chicago, IL, USA). Normality was checked using the Kolmogorov–Smirnov test. Since the data were normally distributed for all continuous parameters tested, mostly parametric methods were used. Descriptive statistics were employed to summarize all variables. Categorical variables are represented as frequencies and percentages, while continuous variables are summarized as means and standard deviations (SDs). All relative rates were calculated using the available data for the variables of interest, and all analyses were conducted following the principles outlined in the Cochrane Handbook [40].

3. Results

In total, we identified 1975 potentially relevant articles in the initial database search. From these, 1941 were excluded following screening, as they were duplicates or not relevant. A total of 34 studies were finally enrolled in this systematic review (Figure 2). Among these, 32 were reports of single cases and 2 were case series, each one including reports of 2 cases. Thorough demographic data of the patients and details of each study are provided in Tables 1 and 2.

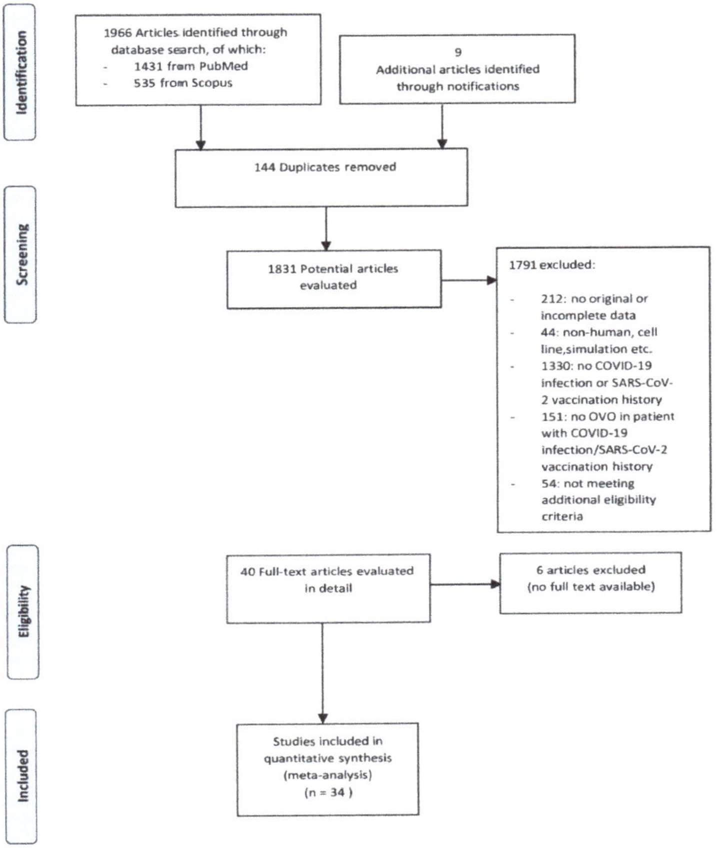

Figure 2. PRISMA Flowchart.

Table 1. Cases of retinal vein occlusion associated with COVID-19 infection or SARS-CoV-2 immunization.

Year, Authors	Age	Sex	Type of Occlusion	Eye	Clinical Symptoms	Time Since COVID-19 Infection or SARS-CoV-2 Immunization (days)	Comorbidities	BCVA at Baseline	Interventions	Final BCVA	Follow-up Period
2020, Gaba et al. [8]	40	Male	CRVO	OU	DV	4 (infection)	Hypertension; Obesity	RE 6/9 LE 6/18	LMWH; Rivaroxaban	RE 6/6 LE 6/12	1 week
2020, Insausti-García et al. [9]	40	Male	CRVO/ Papillophlebitis	OS	DV	42 (infection)	None	20/200	ASA; Bromfenac; Intravitreal dexamethasone implant	20/40	2 weeks

Table 1. *Cont.*

Year, Authors	Age	Sex	Type of Occlusion	Eye	Clinical Symptoms	Time Since COVID-19 Infection or SARS-CoV-2 Immunization (days)	Comorbidities	BCVA at Baseline	Interventions	Final BCVA	Follow-up Period
2020, Rego Lorca et al. [10]	30	Female	CRVO	OU	DV, floaters	N/A (infection)	Maturity-onset DM of the young	BE 7/10	N/A	N/A	N/A
2020, Kapatayes et al. [11]	59	Male	CRVO	OD	DV	N/A (infection)	Microscopic colitis	20/20	None	20/20	N/A
2020, Sheth et al. [12]	52	Male	BRVO	OS	DV	10 (infection)	None	6/60	Oral methylprednisolone; Intravitreal anti-VEGF	6/9	1 month
2020, Walinjkar et al. [13]	17	Female	CRVO	OD	DV	22 (infection)	PCOS	6/24	Intravitreal anti-VEGF	6/18	1 month
2020, Yahalomi et al. [14]	33	Male	CRVO	OS	DV, flashes	35 (infection)	None	20/25	None	20/20	Several months
2021, Finn et al. [15]	32	Male	CRVO	OD	VF defect	N/A (infection)	None	20/20	N/A	N/A	N/A
2021, Raval et al. [16]	39	Male	CRVO	OD	DV, floaters	7 (infection)	None	20/150	Intravitreal anti-VEGF	20/30	N/A
2021, Venkatesh et al. [17]	56	Female	CRVO	OS	DV	N/A (infection)	DM	6/18	Low dose ASA	6/6	1 month
2022, Sugihara et al. [7]	38	Male	BRVO	OS	DV	2 (2nd dose of BNT162b2, Comirnaty, Pfizer-BioNTech vaccine)	None	20/25	Intravitreal anti-VEGF	20/20	7 months
2022, Sonawane et al. [18]	50	Male	CRVO	OD	DV	4 (2nd dose of ChAdOx1 nCoV-19, Covishield, AstraZeneca-Oxford vaccine)	DM	6/60	Intravitreal anti-VEGF	N/A	N/A

Table 1. *Cont.*

Year, Authors	Age	Sex	Type of Occlusion	Eye	Clinical Symptoms	Time Since COVID-19 Infection or SARS-CoV-2 Immunization (days)	Comorbidities	BCVA at Baseline	Interventions	Final BCVA	Follow-up Period
2022, Sonawane et al. [18]	43	Female	CRVO	OD	DV	3 (2nd dose of ChAdOx1 nCoV-19, Covishield, AstraZeneca-Oxford vaccine)	None	5/60	None	N/A	N/A
2022, Cuadros Sánchez et al. [19]	32	Male	CRVO	OD	DV, photopsia	51 (infection)	None	20/32	Intravitreal dexamethasone implant	20/20	4 months
2022, Garduño Vieyra et al. [20]	43	Male	BRVO	OD	DV	4 (infection)	Coats disease	20/400	Intravitreal anti-VEGF; Periocular triamcinolone; Focal laser treatment	20/20	3 months
2022, Pur et al. [21]	34	Male	BRVO	OD	Inferior VF defect, photopsia	2 (1st dose of BNT162b2, Comirnaty, Pfizer-BioNTech vaccine)	None	20/20	None	20/20	10 months
2022, Tanaka et al. [22]	50	Female	BRVO	OD	DV	3 (1st dose of BNT162b2, Comirnaty, Pfizer-BioNTech vaccine)	Breast cancer (treated with tamoxifen)	20/25	Intravitreal anti-VEGF	20/20	2 months
2022, Tanaka et al. [22]	56	Female	BRVO	OD	DV	3 (1st dose of BNT162b2, Comirnaty, Pfizer-BioNTech vaccine)	None	13/20	Intravitreal anti-VEGF	20/20	2 months
2023, Lin et al. [23]	48	Male	CRVO	OU	DV	14 (infection)	Hypertens DM type II; CKD stage IV	OU CF	BE Intravitreal anti-VEGF	OU 20/20	Several months

Table 1. *Cont.*

Year, Authors	Age	Sex	Type of Occlusion	Eye	Clinical Symptoms	Time Since COVID-19 Infection or SARS-CoV-2 Immunization (days)	Comorbidities	BCVA at Baseline	Interventions	Final BCVA	Follow-up Period
2023, Ishiguro et al. [24]	47	Male	CRVO	OD	DV	8 h (1st dose of BNT162b2, Comirnaty, Pfizer-BioNTech vaccine)	None	20/200	Intravitreal anti-VEGF	20/20	10 months
2023, Lee et al. [25]	41	Female	BRVO	OD	Central VF defect	3 (2nd dose of BNT162b2, Comirnaty, Pfizer-BioNTech vaccine)	None	6/18	Intravitreal anti-VEGF	6/6	1 month

BCVA = Best-corrected visual acuity; CRVO = Central retinal vein occlusion; BRVO = Branch retinal vein occlusion; OD = Right eye; OS = Left eye; OU = Both eyes; DV = Decreased vision; VF = Visual field; CF = Counting fingers; DM = Diabetes mellitus; PCOS = Polycystic ovarian syndrome; CKD = Chronic kidney disease; ASA = Acetylsalicylic acid; LMWH = Low molecular weight heparin; VEGF = Vascular endothelial growth factor; N/A = Not available.

Table 2. Cases of retinal artery occlusion associated with COVID-19 infection or SARS-CoV-2 immunization.

Year, Authors	Age	Sex	Type of Occlusion	Eye	Clinical Symptoms	Time Since COVID-19 Infection or SARS-CoV-2 Immunization (days)	Comorbidities	BCVA at Baseline	Interventions	Final BCVA	Follow-up Period
2020, Acharya et al. [6]	60	Male	CRAO	OD	PVL	12 (infection)	Hypertension; Dyslipidemia; Coronary artery disease; COPD	NLP	N/A	NLP	N/A
2020, Montesel et al. [26]	59	Male	CRAO	OS	PVL	21 (infection)	Hypertension; Hyperuricemia; Heterozygous hemoglobin S (sickle cell trait)	LP	None	CF	1 month

Table 2. *Cont.*

Year, Authors	Age	Sex	Type of Occlusion	Eye	Clinical Symptoms	Time Since COVID-19 Infection or SARS-CoV-2 Immunization (days)	Comorbidities	BCVA at Baseline	Interventions	Final BCVA	Follow-up Period
2021, Bapaye et al. [27]	42	Male	CRAO	OU	PVL	13 (infection)	None	OU LP	ASA; Oral dexamethasone	OU LP	6 weeks
2021, Murchison et al. [28]	5th decade	Male	CRAO	OD	PVL	2 (infection)	Hypertension	HM	LMWH	HM	N/A
2021, Raj et al. [29]	37	Male	CRAO	OS	PVL, proptosis, ptosis, ophthalmoplegia	14 (infection)	None	NLP	IV steroids; IV antibiotics; IV anticoagulants; Symptomatic care	NLP	N/A
2021, Sanjay et al. [30]	66	Male	CRAO	OD	PVL	10 (infection)	DM type II	20/2666	Topical prednisolone; Topical anticholinergic	N/A	N/A
2021, Savastano et al. [31]	58	Male	BRAO	OS	None	40 (infection)	Coronary artery disease; Hypertension; Hyperuricemia	55/55	None	55/55	1 week
2021, Turedi et al. [32]	54	Male	CRAO	OD	PVL	14 (infection)	None	CF	Antiglaucoma eye drops; Hyperbaric oxygen therapy; Ocular massage	CF	5 days
2022, Abdin et al. [33]	76	Female	CRAO	OS	PVL	2 (1st dose of ChAdOx1-S [recombinant], Vaxzevria, AstraZeneca-Oxford vaccine)	Hypothyroidism	HM	ASA; IV vasodilator; Antiglaucoma eye drops; Ocular massage	N/A	N/A

Table 2. *Cont.*

Year, Authors	Age	Sex	Type of Occlusion	Eye	Clinical Symptoms	Time Since COVID-19 Infection or SARS-CoV-2 Immunization (days)	Comorbidities	BCVA at Baseline	Interventions	Final BCVA	Follow-up Period
2022, Chow et al. [34]	70	Male	CRAO	OD	PVL	5 (1st dose of mRNA-1273, Spikevax, Moderna vaccine)	Hypertension; Dyslipidemia	CF	Clopidogrel; Hyperbaric oxygen therapy	CF	4 months
2022, Thakar et al. [35]	44	Male	CRAO	OS	PVL	10 (1st dose of BBV152, Covaxin, Bharat Biotech vaccine)	None	LP	None	N/A	N/A
2023, Rv et al. [36]	68	Female	CRAO	OS	PVL	N/A (infection)	Hypertension	20/400	Anti-glaucoma eye drops; Ocular massage;	CF	4 months
2023, Heidarzadeh et al. [37]	44	Male	CRAO	OS	PVL	20 (infection)	None	LP	Oral prednisolone; Anti-glaucoma eye drops; Panretinal photocoagulation	NLP	N/A
2024, Kunihiko et al. [38]	43	Female	BRAO	OD	DV	33 (infection)	None	20/25	IV vasodilator	N/A	6 months
2024, Jiang et al. [39]	76	Male	BRAO	OS	DV	12 (infection)	Hypertension	6/20	ASA; LMWH; Oral prednisolone; IV vasodilator; Retrobulbar anticholinergic; Anterior chamber puncture; Supplemental oxygen	20/20	12 months

BCVA = Best-corrected visual acuity; CRAO = Central retinal artery occlusion; BRAO = Branch retinal artery occlusion; OD = Right eye; OS = Left eye; OU = Both eyes; DV = Decreased vision; PVL = Painless vision loss; DM = Diabetes mellitus; COPD = Chronic obstructive pulmonary disease; NLP = No light perception; LP = Light perception; HM = Hand motion; CF = Counting fingers; ASA = Acetylsalicylic acid; LMWH = Low molecular weight heparin; IV = Intravenous; N/A = Not available.

We further divided retinal vascular occlusion cases into artery (RAO) and vein (RVO) ones. A total of 21 patients (14 males, 66.7%) aged between 17 to 59 years old (mean ± SD = 41.9 ± 10.3 years, Table 1) have been diagnosed with RVO. Among these, 13 cases of retinal vein occlusion (61.9%) occurred after COVID-19 infection, while 8 cases (38.1%) were noted after vaccination. The time to RVO since COVID-19 infection or SARS-CoV-2 immunization ranged from 8 h (1/3 day) to 51 days (mean ± SD = 12.3 ± 15.7 days), with all of the patients complaining about decreased vision or respective visual field defects. The imaging techniques used for the diagnosis of RVO included fundoscopy, optical coherence tomography (OCT), and fluorescein angiography (FA). Nine out of twenty-one patients underwent all three imaging techniques, nine had only fundoscopy and OCT, two patients were examined with fundoscopy and FA, and one patient had only fundoscopic examination available. Twelve out of twenty-one patients were previously healthy, and eight had systemic comorbidities such as obesity, diabetes, hypertension, polycystic ovary syndrome (PCOS), microscopic colitis, chronic kidney disease (CKD), and cancer. One patient had Coats disease as a comorbidity. The laboratory workup showed that six patients had elevated inflammatory markers (6/21, 28.6%) and six patients had elevated coagulation markers (D-dimers, 6/21, 28.6%).

Various treatment modalities were applied to these patients (Figure 3a). One patient was treated with oral methylprednisolone along with intravitreal anti-VEGF injections; one with intravitreal anti-VEGF and periocular triamcinolone injections along with focal laser; nine patients received only intravitreal anti-VEGF injections; one patient was treated with low molecular weight heparin (LMWH) along with rivaroxaban; one was treated only with aspirin; another patient received aspirin, bromfenac eye drops, and an intravitreal dexamethasone implant; another patient was treated only with an intravitreal dexamethasone implant; four patients received no treatment; and for two patients there were no available data. Fifteen out of the twenty-one patients (15/21, 71.4%) had a significant improvement in visual acuity after the resolution of symptoms while two patients maintained their optimal visual acuity both at the onset of retinal vein occlusion and at follow-up. There were no available data for the other four cases.

As far as retinal artery occlusions are concerned, a total of 15 patients (12 males, 80%) aged between 37 to 76 years old (mean ± SD = 56.9 ± 13.2 years, Table 2) have been reported with COVID-19 related RAO. Among these, 12 cases of retinal artery occlusion (80%) occurred after COVID-19 infection, while 3 cases (20%) were reported after vaccination. The time to RAO since COVID-19 infection or SARS-CoV-2 immunization ranged from 2 to 40 days (mean ± SD = 14.9 ± 10.8 days), with the majority of patients (12/15, 80%) complaining of painless vision loss. One patient had no ocular symptoms. The imaging techniques used for diagnosis included fundoscopy, OCT, FA, brain and orbit computed tomography angiography (CTA), head magnetic resonance imaging (MRI), and visually evoked potentials. Six out of the fifteen patients were previously healthy and the other nine had comorbidities such as diabetes, hypertension, dyslipidemia, hyperuricemia, coronary artery disease, chronic obstructive pulmonary disease, hypothyroidism, and sickle cell trait. Six out of the fifteen RAO patients (6/15, 40%) had elevated inflammatory markers, and eight (8/15, 53.3%) did not show improvement. For each patient a different intervention was used (Figure 3b): a combination of aspirin and dexamethasone; LMWH; intravenous (IV) steroids with antibiotics and anticoagulants and symptomatic care; topical prednisolone in a patient with concurrent bilateral panuveitis; ocular massage with hypotensive eye drops; ocular massage with hypotensive eye drops and hyperbaric oxygen therapy; ocular massage with hypotensive eye drops, aspirin, and IV vasodilator; IV vasodilator; clopidogrel and hyperbaric oxygen therapy; a combination of prednisolone and hypotensive eye drops and panretinal photocoagulation; and a combination of aspirin, prednisolone, IV vasodilator, retrobulbar anticholinergic injections, anterior chamber puncture, and supplemental oxygen. Three patients received no treatment and for one patient there were no available data.

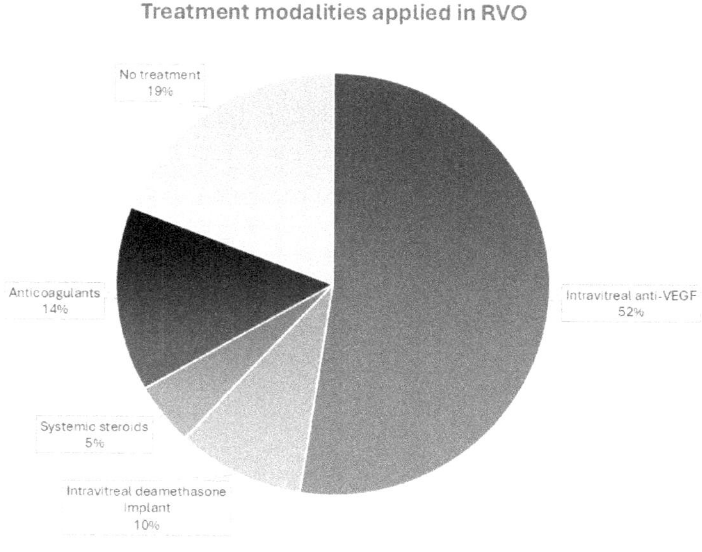

(**a**)

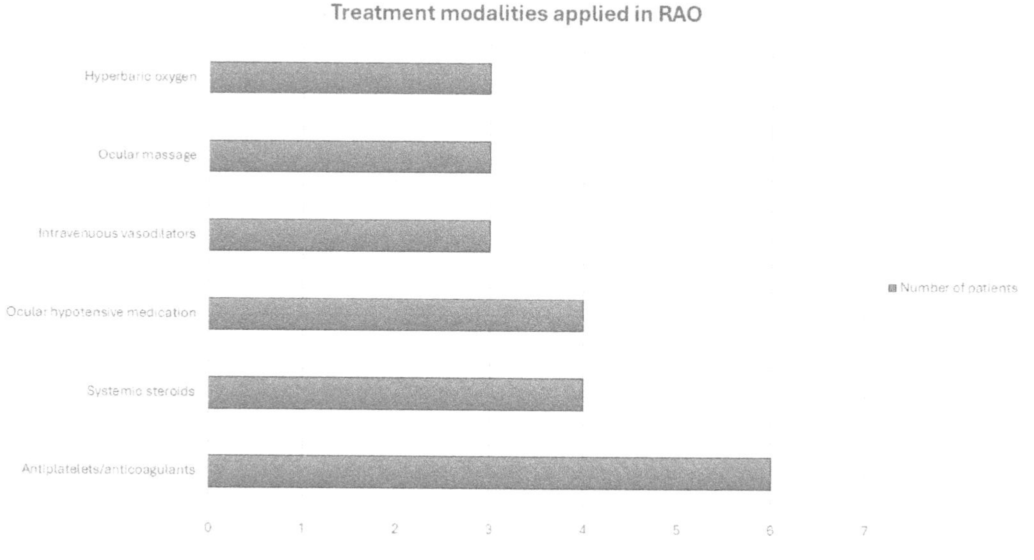

(**b**)

Figure 3. Treatment modalities applied in cases of retinal vein occlusion (RVO, (**a**)), and retinal arterial occlusion (RAO, (**b**)) related to COVID-19 infection or immunization.

4. Discussion

Retinal vascular occlusions are classified among the most common causes of visual loss that occur in people aged >50 years, usually with additional cardiovascular risk factors, such as hypertension and diabetes [4]. CRAO can be either embolic or non-embolic. More commonly, emboli from the heart due to atrial fibrillation and internal carotid artery atherosclerosis lead to acute obstruction of the arterial retinal blood flow, similar to cerebral infarctions. Thus, acute CRAO can lead to irreversible cell death and a permanent decrease in vision within a few hours [5]. A non-embolic way that carotid artery atherosclerosis can cause CRAO is through a significant stenosis of the vessel diameter (>70%), thus reducing the ocular blood flow. Moreover, it is hypothesized that the platelet aggregation in the atherosclerotic plaque results in the release of serotonin, which is a powerful vasoconstrictor and can produce a transient spasm in the retinal arteries [41].

Other non-atherosclerotic causes of CRAO include systemic diseases, such as vasculitis and giant cell arteritis, and hematological diseases such as sickle cell anemia, leukemia, and lymphoma [5]. Autoimmune mediated and infectious disorders, as well as thrombophilia, are also related to CRAO, which has also been reported following hemodialysis and orbital and eye surgery or head injuries [5,41].

Risk factors for central retinal vein occlusion (CRVO) include hypertension, diabetes, glaucoma, and cardiovascular disease [5]. Although the pathogenesis of CRVO is not completely understood, it is considered that the venous obstruction occurs in the region of or most likely just posterior to the lamina cribrosa. It is considered that when the occlusion of the central retinal vein occurs in the lamina cribrosa, it usually causes a more complete obstruction and, therefore, a worse prognosis, while an occlusion posterior to the lamina cribrosa leads to less severe or non-ischemic obstruction [42]. Increased intraocular pressure in particular can displace the lamina cribrosa and change the shape of the central retinal vein, leading to increased turbulence and endothelial stress [5]. Moreover, the central retinal vein can be compressed by a rigid retinal arterial wall, especially in those with atherosclerosis. This occurs because the central retinal artery and vein share a common adventitial sheath [42]. Other predisposing factors include systemic vascular comorbidities and a prothrombotic state [5]. Interestingly, inflammation, dehydration, and exercise can also lead to CRVO in younger people with congenital anomalies but without any other comorbidity [42].

SARS-CoV-2 uses angiotensin-converting-enzyme-2 (ACE-2) receptors to release its RNA inside the host's epithelial cells [43–45]. After the virus has infected the epithelial cells of the lungs, it can enter the bloodstream and travel throughout various parts of the body, including the heart, brain, gastrointestinal tract, kidney, and liver, thus causing symptomatology from the affected organs, such as cerebral hemorrhage and ischemic stroke. Once the virus infects the epithelial cells, it releases cytokines that lead to localized inflammation, endothelial activation, and tissue damage [45]. Zhou et al. have shown that the ACE-2 receptor is also expressed in many non-vascular retinal cells, such as the photoreceptor outer segments, the inner nuclear layer, the inner plexiform layer, and the retinal ganglion cell layer. Furthermore, they observed that there is increased expression of vascular ACE-2 in the retinas of diabetic retinopathy patients [46].

In the case reports that we examined [6–39], around half of RAO and one-third of RVO patients had at least one risk factor, and the remaining patients were individuals without any comorbidity or medication use associated with an increased risk of retinal vascular occlusion. We hypothesize that SARS-CoV-2 infection or immunization, through the release of inflammatory cytokines, has resulted in CRAO or CRVO in patients with other cardiovascular risk factors. Moreover, SARS-CoV-2 may have reached the retinal cells of previously healthy patients, thus causing CRVO and CRAO in younger people through the release of inflammatory cytokines, since inflammation and infectious disorders have already been related to CRVO and CRAO, respectively [5,43,45]. However, further research is essential to understand the link between COVID-19 infection or vaccination and retinal vascular occlusion.

Interestingly, the case of a 58-year-old patient diagnosed with BRAO who did not complain of any symptoms has been reported [17]. This suggests that there may be some subclinical cases of retinal obstruction that go undetected. Another possibility could be that some patients may not be detected because more serious types of thrombosis, such as deep vein thrombosis, mask the presentation of retinal vascular obstruction as a primary clinical concern.

Clinical presentation of COVID-19 related retinal vascular occlusions reviewed in this study did not seem to differ significantly from non-COVID respective cases, as most patients demonstrated decreased vision in vein occlusions and painless vision loss in arterial ones. A male predominance was noticed for both RVO (14/21, 66.7%) and RAO cases (12/15, 80%). Regarding patients' age, patients with COVID-19 related RAO seemed to be older (56.9 $\pm$ 13.2 years old) than patients presenting with vein occlusions during or after their COVID-19 infection or SARS-CoV-2 vaccination (41.9 $\pm$ 10.3 years old) and this difference was found to be statistically significant (Students *t*-test, $p = 0.001$).

Regarding management, several therapeutic modalities have been applied to patients with COVID-related retinal occlusions. The most common among cases reported in this review were anti-VEGF intravitreal injections in vein occlusions, especially in the presence of macular edema, and antiplatelet/anticoagulant medication in arterial ones (Figure 3a,b). The type of treatment, however, did not seem to play a substantial role in terms of visual acuity improvement. The final visual outcome of vein occlusions was much more favorable than that of arterial occlusions, as expected.

Thrombotic complications such as acute limb ischemia due to COVID-19 usually present around 13 days according to one study by Topcu et al. [47], while Fournier et al. estimated the time to presentation at 11 days, with a range of 5 to 20 days [48]. In the case studies included in this review, arterial events in COVID-19 patients and vaccine recipients were detected 2 to 40 days after infection or vaccination (mean $\pm$ SD = 14.9 $\pm$ 10.8 days). Fournier et al. also noted that arterial thrombotic events in COVID-19 seem to be associated with typical cardiovascular risk factors, and that in these patients, mortality is higher [48]. This may be indicative of the assumption that COVID-19 may need "fertile ground" to cause arterial occlusions.

Venous thromboembolism is, similar to arterial events, associated with common risk factors, such as male sex, older age, elevated D-dimers, coronary artery disease, and prior myocardial infarction [49]. It is known that complement activation is increased in COVID-19 patients compared to other causes of pneumonia, suggesting a possible pathophysiologic mechanism implicating local inflammatory responses and the endothelium in venous thrombosis [50–52]. Retinal vein occlusion could also be attributed to comorbidities of the patients included in this study rather than COVID-19 infection or immunization. For instance, Garduno et al. reported on a 43-year-old patient with known Coat's disease who developed BRVO 4 days after testing positive for COVID-19 [20]. These cases with significant risk factors for retinal vein occlusions were not excluded from the analysis as a cause–effect relationship cannot be certain but should be dealt with skepticism.

Another possible "sibling pathology" could be any cerebrovascular complication of COVID-19, due to the common embryologic origin with retinal tissue. Patients with cerebrovascular disease and COVID-19 have worse outcomes than those with non-COVID cerebrovascular disease. This may mean that COVID-19 infection worsens outcomes in patients already at high risk for cerebrovascular complications [53,54]. However, the currently available data does not support any probable pathophysiologic mechanism by which SARS-CoV-2 could cause acute ischemic strokes as a primary culprit [55]. Recently, a multicenter study by Li et al., enrolling more than 1 million COVID-19 patients and controls from 46 healthcare organizations in the United States, demonstrated that people suffering from COVID-19 were more prone to develop branch retinal vein occlusions compared to healthy individuals. The authors concluded that COVID-19 may be associated with retinal vein occlusion, strengthening the results of our study [56].

In conclusion, COVID-19 seems to play a role in the pathogenesis of retinal vascular occlusions, as several cases of RVO and RAO have been reported during or after SARS-CoV-2 infections and vaccinations. Several mechanisms can be proposed by examining various clinical entities with vascular complications associated with COVID-19. However, whether SARS-CoV-2 may be strongly associated with an increased risk of retinal vascular events and the possible pathophysiologic mechanisms have not been fully elucidated. Future studies are expected to shed light on this phenomenon.

Author Contributions: Conceptualization, N.Z. and A.T.; methodology, N.Z., M.G., N.T. and A.T.; software, M.F., M.G. and N.T.; validation, A.T.; formal analysis, A.T., M.F., M.G. and N.T.; investigation, M.F., M.G. and N.T.; resources, N.Z.; data curation, M.F., M.G. and N.T.; writing—original draft preparation, A.T., M.F., M.G. and N.T.; writing—review and editing, N.Z. and A.T.; visualization, M.F.; supervision, N.Z. and A.T. All authors have read and agreed to the published version of the manuscript.

Funding: This research received no external funding.

Institutional Review Board Statement: This study was conducted in accordance with the Declaration of Helsinki and approved by the Institutional Review Board and Ethics Committee of the Aristotle University of Thessaloniki, Papageorgiou General Hospital (ethic approval code: 276/23, ethic approval date: 14 December 2023).

Informed Consent Statement: Informed written consent was waived as no subjects were involved in this study, which is a systematic review.

Data Availability Statement: The raw data supporting this study's findings are available from the corresponding author upon request.

Conflicts of Interest: The authors declare no conflicts of interest.

References

1. Yuki, K.; Fujiogi, M.; Koutsogiannaki, S. COVID-19 pathophysiology: A review. *Clin. Immunol.* **2020**, *215*, 108427. [CrossRef] [PubMed]
2. Gómez-Mesa, J.E.; Galindo-Coral, S.; Montes, M.C.; Martin, A.J.M. Thrombosis and Coagulopathy in COVID-19. *Cur. Probl. Cardiol.* **2021**, *46*, 100742. [CrossRef] [PubMed]
3. Hazar, L.; Karahan, M.; Vural, E.; Ava, S.; Erdem, S.; Dursun, M.E.; Keklikçi, U. Macular vessel density in patients recovered from COVID 19. *Photodiagnosis Photodyn. Ther.* **2021**, *34*, 102267. [CrossRef] [PubMed]
4. Ip, M.; Hendrick, A. Retinal Vein Occlusion Review. *Asia Pac. J. Ophthalmol.* **2018**, *7*, 40–45. [CrossRef]
5. Scott, I.U.; Campochiaro, P.A.; Newman, N.J.; Biousse, V. Retinal vascular occlusions. *Lancet Lond Engl.* **2020**, *396*, 1927–4190. [CrossRef]
6. Acharya, S.; Diamond, M.; Anwar, S.; Glaser, A.; Tyagi, P. Unique case of central retinal artery occlusion secondary to COVID-19 disease. *IDCases* **2020**, *21*, e00867. [CrossRef]
7. Sugihara, K.; Kono, M.; Tanito, M. Branch Retinal Vein Occlusion after Messenger RNA-Based COVID-19 Vaccine. *Case Rep. Ophthalmol.* **2022**, *13*, 28–32. [CrossRef]
8. Gaba, W.H.; Ahmed, D.; Al Nuaimi, R.K.; Dhanhani, A.A.; Eatamadi, H. Bilateral Central Retinal Vein Occlusion in a 40-Year-Old Man with Severe Coronavirus Disease 2019 (COVID-19) Pneumonia. *Am. J. Case Rep.* **2020**, *21*, e927691.29. [CrossRef]
9. Insausti-García, A.; Reche-Sainz, J.A.; Ruiz-Arranz, C.; Vázquez, Á.L.; Ferro-Osuna, M. Papillophlebitis in a COVID-19 patient: Inflammation and hypercoagulable state. *Eur. J. Ophthalmol.* **2020**, *32*, NP168–NP172. [CrossRef]

10. Rego Lorca, D.; Rouco Fernandez, A.; Jimenez Santos, M.; Saenz-Frances, F.; Burgos-Blasco, B.; Donate Lopez, J. Bilateral retinal vein occlusion and diabetic retinopathy after COVID-19. *Acta Ophthalmol.* **2020**, *99*, e1246–e1248. [CrossRef]
11. Kapatayes, N.; Joondeph, B.C. Retinal vein occlusion associated with covid-19. *Retin. Today* **2020**, *2020*, 32–33.
12. Sheth, J.U.; Narayanan, R.; Goyal, J.; Goyal, V. Retinal vein occlusion in COVID-19: A novel entity. *Indian J. Ophthalmol.* **2020**, *68*, 2291–2293. [CrossRef] [PubMed]
13. Walinjkar, J.A.; Makhija, S.C.; Sharma, H.R.; Morekar, S.R.; Natarajan, S. Central retinal vein occlusion with COVID-19 infection as the presumptive etiology. *Indian J. Ophthalmol.* **2020**, *68*, 2572–2574. [CrossRef] [PubMed]
14. Yahalomi, T.; Pikkel, J.; Arnon, R.; Pessach, Y. Central retinal vein occlusion in a young healthy COVID-19 patient: A case report. *Am. J. Ophthalmol. Case Rep.* **2020**, *20*, 100992. [CrossRef]
15. Finn, A.P.; Khurana, R.N.; Chang, L.K. Hemi-retinal vein occlusion in a young patient with COVID-19. *Am. J. Ophthalmol. Case Rep.* **2021**, *22*, 101046. [CrossRef]
16. Raval, N.; Djougarian, A.; Lin, J. Central retinal vein occlusion in the setting of COVID-19 infection. *J. Ophthalmic. Inflamm. Infect.* **2021**, *11*, 10. [CrossRef]
17. Venkatesh, R.; Reddy, N.G.; Agrawal, S.; Pereira, A. COVID-19-associated central retinal vein occlusion treated with oral aspirin. *BMJ Case Rep.* **2021**, *14*, e242987. [CrossRef]
18. Sonawane, N.; Yadav, D.; Kota, A.; Singh, H. Central retinal vein occlusion post-COVID-19 vaccination. *Indian Ophthalmol.* **2022**, *70*, 308. [CrossRef]
19. Cuadros Sánchez, C.; Egüen, C.S.; Gutierrez-Ezquerro, R.; Giralt-Peret, L.; Fonollosa, A. Central Retinal Vein Occlusion Presumably Associated with Lupus Anticoagulant Induced by SARSCoV-2. *Ocul. Immunol. Inflamm.* **2022**, *30*, 2010–2013. [CrossRef]
20. Vieyra, L.G.; Garduño, C.O.; Martínez, R.R.; Escobar, B.F. Branch retinal vein occlusion on Coats disease during COVID-19 infection: A case report. *Oftalmol. Zhurnal* **2022**, *98*, 63–64. [CrossRef]
21. Pur, D.R.; Catherine Danielle Bursztyn, L.L.; Iordanous, Y. Branch retinal vein occlusion in a healthy young man following mRNA COVID-19 vaccination. *Am. J. Ophthalmol. Case Rep.* **2022**, *26*, 101445. [CrossRef] [PubMed]
22. Tanaka, H.; Nagasato, D.; Nakakura, S.; Nagasawa, T.; Wakuda, H.; Kurusu, A.; Mitamura, Y.; Tabuchi, H. Branch retinal vein occlusion post severe acute respiratory syndrome coronavirus 2 vaccination. *Taiwan J. Ophthalmol.* **2022**, *12*, 202. [CrossRef] [PubMed]
23. Lin, C.-H.; Sun, I.-T. Bilateral Simultaneous Central Retinal Vein Occlusion Secondary to COVID-19: A Case Report. *Case Rep Ophthalmol.* **2023**, *14*, 56–61. [CrossRef] [PubMed]
24. Ishiguro, K.; Hirano, Y.; Esaki, Y.; Yasukawa, T. Central Retinal Vein Occlusion after mRNA COVID-19 Vaccination. *Case Rep. Ophthalmol.* **2023**, *14*, 234–240. [CrossRef] [PubMed]
25. Lee, J.; Ong, K.W.; Halim, W.H.M.W.A.; Khialdin, S.M.M.; Yong, M.H.M. Case Report: Branch Retinal Vein Occlusion Post-mRNA SARS-CoV-2 (COVID-19) Vaccination. *Optom. Vis. Sci.* **2023**, *100*, 799–803. [CrossRef]
26. Montesel, A.; Bucolo, C.; Mouvet, V.; Moret, E.; Eandi, C.M. Case Report: Central Retinal Artery Occlusion in a COVID-19 Patient. *Front. Pharmacol.* **2020**, *11*, 588384. [CrossRef]
27. Bapaye, M.M.; Nair, A.G.; Bapaye, C.M.; Shukla, J.J. Simultaneous Bilateral Central Retinal Artery Occlusion Following COVID-19 Infection. *Ocul. Immunol. Inflamm.* **2021**, *29*, 671–674. [CrossRef]
28. Murchison, A.P.; Sweid, A.; Dharia, R.; Theofanis, T.N.; Tjoumakaris, S.I.; Jabbour, P.M.; Bilyk, J.R. Monocular visual loss as the presenting symptom of COVID-19 infection. *Clin. Neurol. Neurosurg.* **2021**, *201*, 106440. [CrossRef]
29. Raj, A.; Kaur, N.; Kaur, N. Cavernous sinus thrombosis with central retinal artery occlusion in COVID-19: A case report and review of literature. *Indian J. Ophthalmol.* **2021**, *69*, 1327–1329. [CrossRef]
30. Sanjay, S.; Srinivasan, P.; Jayadev, C.; Mahendradas, P.; Gupta, A.; Kawali, A.; Shetty, R. Post COVID-19 Ophthalmic Manifestations in an Asian Indian Male. *Ocul. Immunol. Inflamm.* **2021**, *29*, 656–661. [CrossRef]
31. Savastano, M.C.; Culiersi, C.; Savastano, A.; Gambini, G.; Caporossi, T.; Rizzo, S. Focal superior quadrant haemorrhages in post COVID-19 patient: A target for personalized medicine. *Eur. J. Ophthalmol.* **2021**, *32*, NP87–NP91. [CrossRef] [PubMed]
32. Turedi, N.; Onal Gunay, B. Paracentral acute middle maculopathy in the setting of central retinal artery occlusion following COVID-19 diagnosis. *Eur. J. Ophthalmol.* **2021**, *14*, NP62–NP66. [CrossRef]
33. Abdin, A.D.; Gärtner, B.C.; Seitz, B. Central retinal artery occlusion following COVID-19 vaccine administration. *Am. J. Ophthalmol. Case Rep.* **2022**, *26*, 101430. [CrossRef]
34. Chow, S.Y.; Hsu, Y.R.; Fong, V.H. Central retinal artery occlusion after Moderna mRNA-1273 vaccination. *J. Formos. Med. Assoc.* **2022**, *121*, 2369–2370. [CrossRef]
35. Thakar, M.; Bhattacharya, S. Central retinal artery occlusion after vaccination with whole virion inactivated SARSCoV-2 vaccine Covaxin. *Indian J. Ophthalmol.* **2022**, *70*, 3716–3718. [CrossRef] [PubMed]
36. de Oliveira, M.R.; Lucena, A.R.V.; Higino, T.M.; Ventura, C.V. Central retinal artery occlusion with cilioretinal artery sparing secondary to COVID-19: Additional ocular complication. *Indian J. Ophthalmol.* **2023**, *71*, 663–666. [CrossRef] [PubMed]

37. Heidarzadeh, H.R.; Abrishami, M.; Shariati, M.M.; Shahri, S.H.G.; Astaneh, M.R.A. Atypical Central Retinal Artery Occlusion following COVID-19 Infection: A Case Report. *Case Rep. Ophthalmol.* **2023**, *14*, 405–410. [CrossRef]
38. Hirosawa, K.; Inomata, T.; Sung, J.; Morooka, Y.; Huang, T.; Akasaki, Y.; Okumura, Y.; Nagino, K.; Omori, K.; Nakao, S. Unilateral branch retinal artery occlusion in association with COVID-19: A case report. *Int. J. Ophthalmol.* **2024**, *17*, 777–782. [CrossRef]
39. Jiang, Z.; Ji, H.; Zhang, H.; Dong, Z.; Dong, J. Branch retinal artery occlusion in a patient with COVID-19 infection: A case report. *J. Int. Med. Res.* **2024**, *52*, 03000605241284931. [CrossRef]
40. Higgins, J.; Green, S. (Eds.) *Cochrane Handbook for Systematic Reviews of Interventions Version 5.1.0 (Updated March 2011)*; The Cochrane Collaboration: London, UK, 2011.
41. Hayreh, S. Central retinal artery occlusion. *Indian J. Ophthalmol.* **2018**, *66*, 1684. [CrossRef]
42. McAllister, I.L. Central retinal vein occlusion: A review: Central retinal vein occlusion. *Clin. Exp. Ophthalmol.* **2012**, *40*, 48–58. [CrossRef] [PubMed]
43. Noma, H.; Yasuda, K.; Mimura, T.; Ofusa, A.; Shimura, M. Relationship between retinal blood flow and cytokines in central retinal vein occlusion. *BMC Ophthalmol.* **2020**, *20*, 215. [CrossRef] [PubMed]
44. Seah, I.; Agrawal, R. Can the Coronavirus Disease 2019 (COVID-19) Affect the Eyes? A Review of Coronaviruses and Ocular Implications in Humans and Animals. *Ocul. Immunol. Inflamm.* **2020**, *28*, 391–395. [CrossRef]
45. Singh, S.P.; Pritam, M.; Pandey, B.; Yadav, T.P. Microstructure, pathophysiology, and potential therapeutics of COVID-19: A comprehensive review. *J. Med. Virol.* **2021**, *93*, 275–299. [CrossRef]
46. Zhou, T.; Yuan, Z.; Weng, J.; Pei, D.; Du, X.; He, C.; Lai, P. Challenges and advances in clinical applications of mesenchymal stromal cells. *J. Hematol. Oncol.* **2021**, *14*, 24. [CrossRef]
47. Topcu, A.C.; Ozturk-Altunyurt, G.; Akman, D.; Batirel, A.; Demirhan, R. Acute Limb Ischemia in Hospitalized COVID-19 Patients. *Ann. Vasc. Surg.* **2021**, *74*, 88–94. [CrossRef]
48. Fournier, M.; Faille, D.; Dossier, A.; Mageau, A.; Roland, P.N.; Ajzenberg, N.; Borie, R.; Bouadma, L.; Bunel, V.; Castier, Y.; et al. Arterial Thrombotic Events in Adult Inpatients With COVID-19. *Mayo Clin. Proc.* **2021**, *96*, 295–303. [CrossRef]
49. Bilaloglu, S.; Aphinyanaphongs, Y.; Jones, S.; Iturrate, E.; Hochman, J.; Berger, J.S. Thrombosis in Hospitalized Patients With COVID-19 in a New York City Health System. *JAMA* **2020**, *324*, 799–801. [CrossRef]
50. Oncul, S.; Afshar-Kharghan, V. The interaction between the complement system and hemostatic factors. *Curr. Opin. Hematol.* **2020**, *27*, 341–352. [CrossRef]
51. Teuwen, L.-A.; Geldhof, V.; Pasut, A.; Carmeliet, P. COVID-19: The vasculature unleashed. *Nat. Rev. Immunol.* **2020**, *20*, 389–391. [CrossRef]
52. Libby, P.; Lüscher, T. COVID-19 is, in the end, an endothelial disease. *Eur. Heart J.* **2020**, *41*, 3038–3044. [CrossRef] [PubMed]
53. Katsanos, A.H.; Palaiodimou, L.; Zand, R.; Yaghi, S.; Kamel, H.; Navi, B.B.; Turc, G.; Romoli, M.; Sharma, V.K.; Mavridis, D.; et al. The Impact of SARS-CoV-2 on Stroke Epidemiology and Care: A Meta-Analysis. *Ann. Neurol.* **2021**, *89*, 380–388. [CrossRef] [PubMed]
54. Perry, R.J.; Smith, C.J.; Roffe, C.; Simister, R.J.; Narayanamoorthi, S.; Marigold, R.; Willmot, M.; Dixit, A.; Hassan, A.; Quinn, T.J.; et al. Characteristics and outcomes of COVID-19 associated stroke: A UK multicentre case-control study. *J. Neurol. Neurosurg. Psychiatry* **2021**, *92*, 242–248. [CrossRef] [PubMed]
55. Bass, D.I.; Meyer, R.M.; Barros, G.; Carroll, K.T.; Walker, M.; D'Oria, M.; Levitt, M.R. The impact of the COVID-19 pandemic on cerebrovascular disease. *Semin Vasc. Surg.* **2021**, *34*, 20–27. [CrossRef] [PubMed]
56. Li, J.-X.M.; Wei, J.C.-C.; Wang, Y.-H.B.; Bair, H.; Hsu, S.-B.B.; Lin, C.-J. Retinal Vascular Occlusion and COVID-19 Diagnosis: A Multicenter Population-Based Study. *Retina* **2024**, *44*, 345–352. [CrossRef]

Journal of
Clinical Medicine

MDPI

Brief Report

Prevalence and Associations of Epiretinal Membranes in an Elderly English Population: The Bridlington Eye Assessment Project

Craig Wilde [1,2,†], Georgios D. Panos [1,2,*,†], Ali Pooschti [1,2], Hamish K. MacNab [3], Jonathan G. Hillman [3], Stephen A. Vernon [1] and Winfried M. Amoaku [1,2]

1 Division of Ophthalmology and Visual Sciences, School of Medicine, Faculty of Medicine and Health Sciences, University of Nottingham, Nottingham NG7 2UH, UK; craig.wilde@nuh.nhs.uk (C.W.); ali.poostchi2@nuh.nhs.uk (A.P.); profsavernon@doctors.org.uk (S.A.V.); winfried.amoaku@nottingham.ac.uk (W.M.A.)

2 Department of Ophthalmology, Queen's Medical Centre, Nottingham University Hospitals NHS Trust, Nottingham NG7 2UH, UK

3 Medical Centre, Bridlington HU3 2JZ, UK; jghillman@doctors.org.uk (J.G.H.)

* Correspondence: gdpanos@gmail.com; Tel.: +44-115-924-9924

† These authors contributed equally to this work and share first authorship.

Abstract: Purpose: To determine the prevalence and risk factors of epiretinal membranes (ERMs) in an adult English population. **Methods:** The Bridlington Eye Assessment Project is a population-based study of eye disease among residents aged 65 years or older. Comprehensive interviews and ophthalmic examinations were conducted to assess potential risk factors. Digital mydriatic nonstereoscopic 30° colour fundus photography (CFP) was performed. ERMs were classified as primary/idiopathic or secondary on the basis of findings from the ocular examination and the structured questionnaire. Logistic regression models were used to determine the independence of potential risk factors for idiopathic ERMs. **Results:** In a comprehensive screening of 3588 patients aged over 65, we identified an eye-based prevalence of ERMs of 4.26% and a subject-based prevalence of ERMs of 6.88%. The majority of these cases were idiopathic in nature (90.7%), while 9.3% were secondary ERMs; predominantly, there was a history of cataract surgery (43.5%). No significant correlation between idiopathic ERMs and factors such as age, gender, diabetes, hypertension, a history of stroke, or the presence of AMD was found. **Conclusions:** The prevalence of ERMs in an elderly English population and the proportion of idiopathic and secondary ERMs are similar to previous reports. However, in elderly patients aged over 65 years, age is not a risk factor for the presence of idiopathic ERMs. The presence of diabetes, hypertension, a history of stroke, and AMD of any grade was not associated with ERMs.

Keywords: epiretinal membrane; ERM; prevalence; risk factors; ageing; hypertension; diabetes; stroke; English population; European population

1. Introduction

Epiretinal membranes (ERMs) are a common retinal condition among the elderly. Although mostly asymptomatic, they can lead to a significant loss of visual acuity, cause visual symptoms such as distortion and metamorphopsia, and negatively impact the quality of life [1–3]. They may occur in the absence of any comorbid ocular pathology other than posterior vitreous detachment (PVD), where they are termed idiopathic or primary ERMs [4]. Secondary ERMs are those associated with other ocular diseases, including previous intraocular surgery, various retinal pathologies including retinal breaks and detachments, retinal vein occlusions, diabetic retinopathy, retinitis pigmentosa, previous retinal laser/cryopexy, and uveitis [5].

The Beaver Dam Eye Study (BDES) was the first population-based report of ERM prevalence in 1994 [6]. Since then, many other large population studies have reported the epidemiology of ERMs, mostly utilising colour fundus photography (CFP); however, the more recent studies have additionally used spectral domain optical coherence tomography (SDOCT) [7,8]. These studies, across different ethnicities and geographical regions, demonstrate great heterogeneity in ERM prevalence, including 1% in a Chinese population and 18.5% among Latinos [9,10]. The reasons for such variation are likely complex and may relate to the study design, population demographics such as the age range, as well as the grading methodology and imaging techniques. A recent systematic review and meta-analysis of population-based studies concluded that in specific regions, including Europe, robust evidence for prevalence and risk factors for ERMs remains absent, with most studies included being carried out in the Pacific Rim nations of the USA, Australia, Japan, Singapore, and China [11]. Although it could be argued that many of these already include large Caucasian populations of European ancestry, it is possible that true ethnic and population variations exist and relate to genetic predispositions, lifestyle factors including smoking, or clinical comorbidities such as diabetes, which vary between countries [6,12]. Interestingly, in the Melbourne Collaborative Cohort Study, among an older Australian population, the prevalence of ERMs was almost twice as high in participants of Southern European origin compared to those of Northern European ancestry [13]. It could be argued that Southern Europeans have a more pigmented fundus when compared to their Northern European counterparts, and ERMs are subsequently more easily detectable. However, the difference in pigmentation does not seem adequate to explain the result. While some other studies report higher prevalence rates among subjects with more pigmented skin, such as the Singapore Indian Eye Study (SINDI) (10.5%) and the Los Angeles Latino Eye Study (LALES) (18.5%), others have reported lower prevalence measures than the largest Caucasian studies [14,15]. Examples include the Beijing Eye Study in China (2.2%) and the Funagata study in Japan (5.44%) [16,17]. On the other hand, a recent study on vitreoretinal interface changes in Ghanaian Africans reported an ERM prevalence of 13.2% (eye-based) [18].

To date, there are two European studies that report ERM prevalence among European populations. However, the UK Biobank study reports prevalence among a 25% subsample of subjects, all of whom have visual impairment, and is not representative of the general UK population [19]. The Maastricht Study in the Netherlands did not recruit patients randomly or consecutively from within their population. Subjects were recruited following media campaigns for volunteers and from various registries, including a regional diabetes patient registry. The study stratified recruitment according to known type 2 diabetes mellitus, with an oversampling of individuals with diabetes [20].

To address the paucity of data among European populations, we aimed to describe the prevalence of ERMs and associated risk factors in an adult English population using data from the Bridlington Eye Assessment Project (BEAP).

2. Materials and Methods

2.1. Study Population

The BEAP is a single-centre population-based study in East Yorkshire, England, aimed at assessing the efficacy of eye disease screening in a population aged 65 and over. The approach utilised clinical assessments conducted by trained optometrists alongside digital imaging technology. The principal ocular conditions investigated were age-related macular degeneration (AMD), cataracts, and glaucoma. An exhaustive description of the study's design and methodology has been detailed in previous publications [21,22]. In summary, all permanent residents aged $\geq$65 years registered with the town's only GP practice were invited to attend by letter on a street-by-street basis. Patients registered as blind, bed-bound, or known to have significant dementia were excluded from the study. The Scarborough and North Yorkshire Local Ethics Research Committee approved the study protocol (Ref No. PB/RH/02/288), and the study was conducted according to the recommendations of the Declaration of Helsinki. Study recruitment occurred between 5 November 2002 and 29 March 2006.

2.2. Interview and Examination Procedures

A trained research nurse conducted in-person interviews with all participants, employing a structured questionnaire to gather demographic details and information pertaining to their ophthalmic and medical histories, including diabetes, previous strokes, and hypertension. Specific histories of previous ophthalmic surgeries, diabetic retinopathy, glaucoma, and macular degeneration were sought.

LogMAR VA was recorded for each eye corrected with both current glasses or contact lenses and a pinhole (Baylie Lovie no. 4 chart). A full biomicroscopic ophthalmic examination was then performed, including grading of lens status (LOCS III), intraocular pressure, central corneal thickness, and the presence of pseudophakia, which were documented during the slit lamp examination. A dilated fundus examination was performed using a 90D lens (Volk Optical, Mentor, OH, USA) by one of four specially trained optometrists. The findings were documented on a structured proforma by research staff, who maintained anonymity in the data recording process. A digital nonstereoscopic CFP was conducted using a fundus camera (model TRC NWS, Topcon, Tokyo, Japan) equipped with a 10-megapixel camera back (Nikon, Tokyo, Japan). For each eye, a single 30-degree field focused on the macula (corresponding to the Early Treatment for Diabetic Retinopathy Study standard field 2) was captured. In cases where the initial images were deemed unsatisfactory, they were promptly retaken.

2.3. Grading of Retinal Photographs

The methodology for grading macular pathology, specifically AMD, and the quality control and adjudication procedures, including assessments of intergrader reliability, have been detailed in a previous publication [23]. All fundus photographs were assessed in a masked fashion by a single ophthalmologist who had received training in image grading using standard definitions and grids as described by the International Classification System for AMD [24]. No medical records or subject demographic data were available during the grading process. Images were graded for macular ERMs using a grid with an outer diameter of 3000 μm, which was placed over the image during grading. No enhancement tools were used for the grading of ERMs. Epiretinal membranes were identified in keeping with the original definitions as used in the BDES [7] and were recorded as present if there was a patch or patches of irregular increased reflection from the inner retinal surface giving a 'glinting, water-silk, and shifting light reflex' without retinal folds or the presence of a more opaque and grey appearance on the inner retinal surface with superficial retinal folds or traction lines. ERMs outside the grid were graded as absent.

2.4. Classification of ERM

ERMs were classified as primary/idiopathic or secondary on the basis of findings from the ocular examination and the structured questionnaire after data merging. Primary ERMs were recorded if no cause for ERM development was evident. Secondary ERMs were defined as those occurring in the eyes in the presence of ocular comorbidities, including previous retinal detachment or retinal tear, previous retinal laser or cryopexy, retinal vascular disease, previous cataract surgery, and diabetic retinopathy [6,25].

2.5. Definitions

In the context of this study, the diagnosis of diabetes mellitus was based on either a self-reported history of diagnosis by a physician or the receipt of drug treatment, including insulin or oral hypoglycaemic agents. Hypertension was identified through a self-reported history of diagnosis by a physician, the use of medication for hypertension, or the presence of elevated blood pressure observed during clinical measurements (systolic blood pressure $\geq$ 140 mmHg or diastolic blood pressure $\geq$ 90 mmHg).

2.6. Statistical Analysis

Data obtained from the grading process were inputted and subjected to internal quality control checks, with any identified discrepancies subsequently corrected. Statistical analysis was performed using MedCalc Statistical Software version 18.2.1 (MedCalc Software bv, Ostend, Belgium) and Jamovi version 2.4 (The Jamovi Project (2023), https://www.jamovi.org accessed on 15 December 2023). The prevalence of ERMs was determined by calculating the percentage of the total population in which cases were identified in either one or both eyes. For idiopathic ERMs, logistic regression models were used to determine the independence of potential risk factors. Potential associations included age, gender (female), history of stroke (yes or no), diabetes (present or absent), and hypertension (present or absent). Odds ratios (OR) and 95% confidence intervals (CI) were calculated. p-values less than 0.05 were deemed to indicate statistical significance. The goodness of fit of the logistic regression model was evaluated using the Hosmer–Lemeshow test. Additionally, a logistic mixed model, accounting for within-subject correlation, was used to determine the association between AMD and ERMs.

3. Results

In total, 3588 patients aged over 65 years old were screened, of whom 2017 were female (56.2% female and 43.8% male). The mean age ± SD of the patients was 74.3 ± 6.6 years. ERMs were detected in CFP in 306 eyes (eye-based prevalence of 4.26%) from 247 subjects (subject-based prevalence of 6.88%). Idiopathic ERMs were found in 224 patients (90.7%) and secondary ERMs in 23 patients (9.3%). A summary of the results is depicted in Table 1.

Table 1. A summary of the results of the study.

Total number of patients	3588
Age (mean ± SD)	74.3 ± 6.6 years
Gender distribution	2016 (56.2%) female, 1572 (43.8%) male
Eye-based ERM prevalence	4.26%
Subject-based ERM prevalence	6.88%
Idiopathic ERM	224 (90.7%)
Secondary ERM	23 (9.3%)

The patients diagnosed with ERMs had a mean age of 75.1 ± 5.25 years. The BCVA for these patients, calculated on an eye-based analysis, was recorded at 0.26 logMAR ± 0.57. Regarding the gender distribution among ERM patients, there were 127 females and 120 males. In terms of associated health conditions, 22 of the ERM patients were identified as having diabetes. A significant number of patients, 122 in total, were found to have hypertension, and 19 patients had a history of stroke. Additionally, our data showed that among the ERM patients, 49 had dry AMD, while 2 patients were identified with wet AMD.

Table 2 illustrates a comprehensive summary of the characteristics of patients with ERMs.

Logistic regression analysis failed to show a correlation between the presence of idiopathic ERMs and factors such as age, gender (female), diabetes, hypertension, and a history of stroke (see Table 3). Among the 23 cases (9.3%) with secondary ERMs, the most frequent cause was a history of cataract surgery, accounting for 43.5% (10 out of 23). The model was a good fit for the data (Hosmer–Lemeshow test, $p = 0.77$). Moreover, there was no evidence of an association between ERMs and any AMD grade (all $p > 0.05$, Table 4).

Table 2. A summary of the ERM patients' characteristics.

Characteristic	Data
Mean age (years)	75.1 ± 5.25
Mean best corrected visual acuity (logMAR)	0.26 ± 0.57
Gender distribution	
-Female	127 (51.4%)
-Male	120 (48.6%)
Patients with diabetes	22 (8.9%)
Patients with hypertension	122 (49.4%)
Patients with stroke	19 (7.7%)
Patients with dry AMD	49 (19.8%)
Patients with wet AMD	2 (0.8%)

Table 3. Results of the logistic regression analysis.

Factor	Coefficient	Std. Error	Wald	Odds Ratio	95% CI	p
Age	0.013612	0.010315	1.7415	1.0137	0.9934 to 1.0344	*0.1869*
Gender (female)	−0.22238	0.13274	2.8064	0.8006	0.6172 to 1.0385	*0.0939*
Diabetes	−0.12292	0.23350	0.2772	0.8843	0.5596 to 1.3976	*0.5986*
Hypertension	−0.084716	0.13579	0.3892	0.9188	0.7041 to 1.1989	*0.5327*
Stroke	−0.20336	0.24978	0.6629	0.8160	0.5001 to 1.3314	*0.4155*

Table 4. Relationship between ERMs and AMD (logistic mixed model).

	Odds Ratio	95% CI	p
Dry AMD	1.80	0.0207 to 157	*0.797*
Geographic atrophy	0	-	*1.0*
Neovascular AMD	6.00×10^{-10}	2.83×10^{-226} to 1.28×10^{207}	*0.978*

4. Discussion

Our investigation into the prevalence and risk factors associated with ERMs in an elderly population offers a comprehensive global perspective, enriched by comparisons with findings from a diverse array of international studies. Our study, revealing an eye-based prevalence of 4.26% and a subject-based prevalence of 6.88%, presents a striking contrast to other studies. Notably, the Handan Eye Study reported a prevalence of 3.4% in a rural Chinese cohort, markedly lower than rates observed in other Asian populations and Caucasian groups [26]. This disparity in prevalence rates across different ethnicities, as also seen in the LALES, Melbourne Collaborative Cohort Study (MCCS), SINDI, and Singapore Malay Eye Study (SiMES), underscores the possible significant influence of ethnic and racial factors on ERM prevalence [13–15,27]. Contrary to findings from other studies where age emerged as a predominant risk factor, our study did not identify age as a significant factor, likely due to the exclusive focus on an elderly cohort over 65 years old. Previous research has indicated that the prevalence of ERMs increases with age until 75 years [6]. Given that the mean age in our study was 74.3 years, this aligns with the notion that beyond this age threshold, age may not be a primary risk factor. Furthermore, this finding is similar to the absence of age correlation in the recent report from Ghana [18]. Additionally, it is also plausible that the presence of cataracts can obscure the detection of very mild ERMs when using direct ophthalmoscopy or fundus photography. This oversight might contribute, at least in part, to underestimating the presence of ERMs in older patients, thereby potentially influencing the perceived lack of correlation between age and ERM risk. This also suggests that, within the older age group, other factors may play a more crucial role in the development of ERMs. Moreover, unlike several other studies, female gender was not identified as a risk factor in our study. This could be attributed to the specific demographic and health characteristics of our elderly cohort, where gender-related differences in ocular health might be less pronounced or overshadowed by age-related changes and comorbidities. This absence of gender correlation with vitreomacular interface changes is similar to that in the recent report from Ghana [18]. Furthermore, our findings indicate that the presence of diabetes, hypertension, and a history of stroke were not associated with ERMs. These results are particularly noteworthy as they contrast with common assumptions about these systemic conditions as risk factors for ocular diseases. Our study also found that AMD of any grade was not correlated with ERMs, a finding that aligns with the results of the Ghana AMD Study Group [18]. This consistency across different studies and populations suggests a more complex relationship between AMD and vitreoretinal interface changes than previously understood [28–30], potentially influenced by factors other than those commonly associated with AMD.

While increasing age was a consistent risk factor in most studies, the Handan Eye Study's association of myopia with primary ERMs aligns with findings from the Visual Impairment Project (VIP) Study [26,31]. Intriguingly, an inverse association between current smoking and primary ERMs was observed in the Handan Eye Study, paralleling reports from the VIP and SiMES [26,27,31]. This could suggest a protective effect of smoking or a survival bias among smokers, a hypothesis warranting further exploration. The methodological choices, particularly the use of OCT versus CFP, significantly impact ERM detection and prevalence estimation. The Handan Eye Study's integration of OCT with retinal photographic diagnosis likely reduced the underestimation of ERM prevalence, highlighting the critical role of diagnostic methodologies in epidemiological research [26]. The SiMES and SINDI studies, focusing on Malay and Indian populations in Singapore, reported higher ERM prevalence rates compared to Caucasian populations, challenging previous assumptions about lower ERM prevalence in Asian groups [14,27]. These findings, along with the higher prevalence observed in the LALES among Latinos, suggest a complex interplay of genetic, environmental, and lifestyle factors influencing ERM development across different ethnicities [15]. Our study, along with international comparisons, underscores the need for heightened clinical awareness and targeted screening strategies for ERMs, particularly in ageing populations. The varying prevalence rates and risk factor associations across different ethnicities and regions highlight the importance of culturally tailored public health interventions and eye care services. While our study and international comparisons provide valuable insights, they also reveal limitations, such as potential residual confounding and variations in diagnostic criteria and methodologies. Notably, our study's lack of OCT examinations is a significant limitation. Although CFP, our employed method, is a gold-standard technique and our study's results are comparable to most previous studies, the inclusion of OCT would have provided much higher sensitivity, crucial for detecting subtle retinal changes. Additionally, the absence of refractive error and axial length measurements in our study represents another limitation. These measurements are important for understanding the development and progression of ocular conditions, and their omission could impact the comprehensiveness of our findings.

Future research should focus on longitudinal studies to elucidate causal relationships, explore any possible genetic underpinnings of ERMs, and assess the impact of lifestyle factors such as diet and smoking. Additionally, advancements in imaging technologies (including OCT) would refine the detection and classification of ERMs, enhancing our understanding of their epidemiology and pathophysiology. A detailed future study exploring the longitudinal relationship between the vitreoretinal interface and the development of a posterior vitreous detachment and association with ERMs would be invaluable. Localised anatomical considerations, such as axial length and refractive status variations, would be useful future considerations in population studies.

In conclusion, our study, enriched by global comparisons, contributes significantly to the existing literature on ERM prevalence, highlighting the importance of methodological consistency, demographic considerations, and the need for ongoing research to elucidate the incidence and risk factors of ERMs in diverse populations and ethnic groups with a particular emphasis on age-specific cohorts and the nuanced role of gender.

Author Contributions: All authors participated in data collection, writing, and editing the manuscript. G.D.P. and C.W. contributed equally and share first authorship. G.D.P. conducted the statistical analysis. All authors have read and agreed to the published version of the manuscript.

Funding: The Bridlington Eye Assessment Project was funded by an unrestricted grant from Pfizer. We would also like to thank the following organisations for their financial support of the project: Pharmacia, Yorkshire Wolds and Coast Primary Care Trust, the Lords Feoffees of Bridlington, Bridlington Hospital League of Friends, the Hull and East Riding Charitable Trust, the National Eye Research Centre (Yorkshire), the Rotary Club of Bridlington, the Alexander Pigott Wernher Memorial Trust, Bridlington Lions Club, the Inner Wheel Club of Bridlington, Soroptimist International of Bridlington, and The Patricia and Donald Shepherd Charitable Trust.

Institutional Review Board Statement: The study received approval from the local ethics committee (Scarborough and North-East Yorkshire Local Ethics Research Committee; Ref No. PB/RH/02/288), and its methodology adhered to the tenets of the Declaration of Helsinki.

Informed Consent Statement: Informed consent was obtained from all participants involved in the study.

Data Availability Statement: The data presented in this study are available on request from the corresponding author.

Acknowledgments: This research was funded in part by a research grant from the Macular Society UK, Andover, Hants, UK.

Conflicts of Interest: The authors report no conflicts of interest and have no proprietary interest in any of the materials mentioned in this article. The funders had no role in the design of the study; in the collection, analyses, or interpretation of data; in the writing of the manuscript; or in the decision to publish the results.

References

1. Scott, I.U.; Smiddy, W.E.; Merikansky, A.; Feuer, W. Vitreoretinal Surgery Outcomes. Impact on Bilateral Visual Function. *Ophthalmology* **1997**, *104*, 1041–1048. [CrossRef] [PubMed]
2. Bouwens, M.D.; Van Meurs, J.C. Sine Amsler Charts: A New Method for the Follow-up of Metamorphopsia in Patients Undergoing Macular Pucker Surgery. *Graefes Arch. Clin. Exp. Ophthalmol.* **2003**, *241*, 89–93. [CrossRef] [PubMed]
3. Okamoto, F.; Okamoto, Y.; Fukuda, S.; Hiraoka, T.; Oshika, T. Vision-Related Quality of Life and Visual Function after Vitrectomy for Various Vitreoretinal Disorders. *Investig. Ophthalmol. Vis. Sci.* **2010**, *51*, 744–751. [CrossRef] [PubMed]
4. Englmaier, V.A.; Storp, J.J.; Dierse, S.; Eter, N.; Al-Nawaiseh, S. Idiopathic Epiretinal Membranes–Pathophysiology, Classifications and Oct-Biomarkers. *Klin. Monbl. Augenheilkd.* 2023; *epub ahead of print*.
5. Ozog, M.K.; Nowak-Was, M.; Rokicki, W. Pathophysiology and Clinical Aspects of Epiretinal Membrane–Review. *Front. Med.* **2023**, *10*, 1121270. [CrossRef] [PubMed]
6. Klein, R.; Klein, B.E.; Wang, Q.; Moss, S.E. The Epidemiology of Epiretinal Membranes. *Trans. Am. Ophthalmol. Soc.* **1994**, *92*, 403–425; discussion 25–30. [PubMed]
7. Meuer, S.M.; Myers, C.E.; Klein, B.E.; Swift, M.K.; Huang, Y.; Gangaputra, S.; Pak, J.W.; Danis, R.P.; Klein, R. The Epidemiology of Vitreoretinal Interface Abnormalities as Detected by Spectral-Domain Optical Coherence Tomography: The Beaver Dam Eye Study. *Ophthalmology* **2015**, *122*, 787–795. [CrossRef] [PubMed]
8. Ye, H.; Zhang, Q.; Liu, X.; Cai, X.; Yu, W.; Yu, S.; Wang, T.; Lu, W.; Li, X.; Hu, Y.; et al. Prevalence and Associations of Epiretinal Membrane in an Elderly Urban Chinese Population in China: The Jiangning Eye Study. *Br. J. Ophthalmol.* **2015**, *99*, 1594–1597. [CrossRef] [PubMed]
9. Zhu, X.F.; Peng, J.J.; Zou, H.D.; Fu, J.; Wang, W.W.; Xu, X.; Zhang, X. Prevalence and Risk Factors of Idiopathic Epiretinal Membranes in Beixinjing Blocks, Shanghai, China. *PLoS ONE* **2012**, *7*, e51445. [CrossRef] [PubMed]
10. Fraser-Bell, S.; Guzowski, M.; Rochtchina, E.; Wang, J.J.; Mitchell, P. Five-Year Cumulative Incidence and Progression of Epiretinal Membranes: The Blue Mountains Eye Study. *Ophthalmology* **2003**, *110*, 34–40. [CrossRef] [PubMed]
11. Xiao, W.; Chen, X.; Yan, W.; Zhu, Z.; He, M. Prevalence and Risk Factors of Epiretinal Membranes: A Systematic Review and Meta-Analysis of Population-Based Studies. *BMJ Open* **2017**, *7*, e014644. [CrossRef] [PubMed]
12. Mitchell, P.; Smith, W.; Chey, T.; Wang, J.J.; Chang, A. Prevalence and Associations of Epiretinal Membranes. The Blue Mountains Eye Study, Australia. *Ophthalmology* **1997**, *104*, 1033–1040. [CrossRef]

13. Aung, K.Z.; Makeyeva, G.; Adams, M.K.; Chong, E.W.; Busija, L.; Giles, G.G.; English, D.R.; Hopper, J.; Baird, P.N.; Guymer, R.H.; et al. The Prevalence and Risk Factors of Epiretinal Membranes: The Melbourne Collaborative Cohort Study. *Retina* **2013**, *33*, 1026–1034. [CrossRef] [PubMed]
14. Koh, V.; Cheung, C.Y.; Wong, W.L.; Cheung, C.M.; Wang, J.J.; Mitchell, P.; Younan, C.; Saw, S.M.; Wong, T.Y. Prevalence and Risk Factors of Epiretinal Membrane in Asian Indians. *Investig. Ophthalmol. Vis. Sci.* **2012**, *53*, 1018–1022. [CrossRef] [PubMed]
15. Fraser-Bell, S.; Ying-Lai, M.; Klein, R.; Varma, R.; Los Angeles Latino Eye Study Group. Prevalence and Associations of Epiretinal Membranes in Latinos: The Los Angeles Latino Eye Study. *Investig. Ophthalmol. Vis. Sci.* **2004**, *45*, 1732–1736. [CrossRef] [PubMed]
16. You, Q.; Xu, L.; Jonas, J.B. Prevalence and Associations of Epiretinal Membranes in Adult Chinese: The Beijing Eye Study. *Eye* **2008**, *22*, 874–879. [CrossRef] [PubMed]
17. Kawasaki, R.; Wang, J.J.; Sato, H.; Mitchell, P.; Kato, T.; Kawata, S.; Kayama, T.; Yamashita, H.; Wong, T.Y. Prevalence and Associations of Epiretinal Membranes in an Adult Japanese Population: The Funagata Study. *Eye* **2009**, *23*, 1045–1051. [CrossRef] [PubMed]
18. Amoaku, W.M.; Cushley, L.; Silvestri, V.; Akafo, S.; Amissah-Arthur, K.N.; Lartey, S.; Hageman, C.N.; Pappas, C.M.; Hubbard, W.C.; Bernstein, P.S.; et al. Vitreomacular Interface Abnormalities in the Ghanaian African. *Eye*, 2023, *ahead of print*. [CrossRef]
19. McKibbin, M.; Farragher, T.; Shickle, D. Vitreoretinal Interface Abnormalities in Middle-Aged Adults with Visual Impairment in the Uk Biobank Study: Prevalence, Impact on Visual Acuity and Associations. *BMJ Open Ophthalmol.* **2017**, *1*, e000057. [CrossRef] [PubMed]
20. Liesenborghs, I.; De Clerck, E.E.B.; Berendschot, T.; Goezinne, F.; Schram, M.T.; Henry, R.M.A.; Stehouwer, C.D.A.; Webers, C.A.B.; Schouten, J. Prevalence of Optical Coherence Tomography Detected Vitreomacular Interface Disorders: The Maastricht Study. *Acta Ophthalmol.* **2018**, *96*, 729–735. [CrossRef] [PubMed]
21. Wilde, C.; Poostchi, A.; Panos, G.D.; Hillman, J.G.; MacNab, H.K.; Dua, H.; Amoaku, W.M.; Vernon, S.A. Prevalence of Reduced Vision among Uk Elderly Drivers: The Bridlington Eye Assessment Project (Beap)-a Cross-Sectional Study. *J. Ophthalmol.* **2022**, *2022*, 8321948. [CrossRef]
22. Vernon, S.A.; Hillman, J.G.; Macnab, H.K.; Bacon, P.; van der Hoek, J.; Vernon, O.K.; Bhargarva, A. Community Optometrist Referral of Those Aged 65 and over for Raised Iop Post-Nice: Aop Guidance Versus Joint College Guidance--an Epidemiological Model Using Beap. *Br. J. Ophthalmol.* **2011**, *95*, 1534–1536. [CrossRef] [PubMed]
23. Wilde, C.; Poostchi, A.; Mehta, R.L.; MacNab, H.K.; Hillman, J.G.; Vernon, S.A.; Amoaku, W.M. Prevalence of Age-Related Macular Degeneration in an Elderly Uk Caucasian Population-the Bridlington Eye Assessment Project: A Cross-Sectional Study. *Eye* **2017**, *31*, 1042–1050. [CrossRef]
24. Bird, A.C.; Bressler, N.M.; Bressler, S.B.; Chisholm, I.H.; Coscas, G.; Davis, M.D.; de Jong, P.T.; Klaver, C.C.; Klein, B.E.; Klein, R.; et al. An International Classification and Grading System for Age-Related Maculopathy and Age-Related Macular Degeneration. The International Arm Epidemiological Study Group. *Surv. Ophthalmol.* **1995**, *39*, 367–374. [CrossRef]
25. Appiah, A.P.; Hirose, T. Secondary Causes of Premacular Fibrosis. *Ophthalmology* **1989**, *96*, 389–392. [CrossRef] [PubMed]
26. Duan, X.R.; Liang, Y.B.; Friedman, D.S.; Sun, L.P.; Wei, W.B.; Wang, J.J.; Wang, G.L.; Liu, W.; Tao, Q.S.; Wang, N.L.; et al. Prevalence and Associations of Epiretinal Membranes in a Rural Chinese Adult Population: The Handan Eye Study. *Investig. Ophthalmol. Vis. Sci.* **2009**, *50*, 2018–2023. [CrossRef] [PubMed]
27. Kawasaki, R.; Wang, J.J.; Mitchell, P.; Aung, T.; Saw, S.M.; Wong, T.Y.; Group Singapore Malay Eye Study. Racial Difference in the Prevalence of Epiretinal Membrane between Caucasians and Asians. *Br. J. Ophthalmol.* **2008**, *92*, 1320–1324. [CrossRef] [PubMed]
28. Lee, S.J.; Koh, H.J. Effects of Vitreomacular Adhesion on Anti-Vascular Endothelial Growth Factor Treatment for Exudative Age-Related Macular Degeneration. *Ophthalmology* **2011**, *118*, 101–110. [CrossRef] [PubMed]
29. Krebs, I.; Brannath, W.; Glittenberg, C.; Zeiler, F.; Sebag, J.; Binder, S. Posterior Vitreomacular Adhesion: A Potential Risk Factor for Exudative Age-Related Macular Degeneration? *Am. J. Ophthalmol.* **2007**, *144*, 741–746. [CrossRef] [PubMed]
30. Lee, S.J.; Lee, C.S.; Koh, H.J. Posterior Vitreomacular Adhesion and Risk of Exudative Age-Related Macular Degeneration: Paired Eye Study. *Am. J. Ophthalmol.* **2009**, *147*, 621–626.e1. [PubMed]
31. McCarty, D.J.; Mukesh, B.N.; Chikani, V.; Wang, J.J.; Mitchell, P.; Taylor, H.R.; McCarty, C.A. Prevalence and Associations of Epiretinal Membranes in the Visual Impairment Project. *Am. J. Ophthalmol.* **2005**, *140*, 288–294. [CrossRef] [PubMed]

MDPI AG
Grosspeteranlage 5
4052 Basel
Switzerland
Tel.: +41 61 683 77 34

Journal of Clinical Medicine Editorial Office
E-mail: jcm@mdpi.com
www.mdpi.com/journal/jcm

www.ingramcontent.com/pod-product-compliance
Lightning Source LLC
Chambersburg PA
CBHW062106220926
51850CB00010B/2908
* 9 7 8 3 7 2 5 8 5 8 5 3 8 *